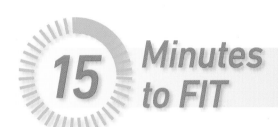

15 Minutes to FIT

15 Minutes to FIT

The Simple 30-Day Guide to Total Fitness, 15 Minutes at a Time

ZUZKA LIGHT and JEFF O'CONNELL

AVERY

an imprint of Penguin Random House

New York

an imprint of Penguin Random House LLC
375 Hudson Street
New York, New York 10014

Copyright © 2015 by Zuzka Light

Exercise photos by Klaudia Seidl
Recipe photos by Zuzka Light
Lifestyle photos by Ashley Erin Dean

Most Avery books are available at special quantity discounts for bulk purchase for sales promotions, premiums, fund-raising, and educational needs. Special books or book excerpts also can be created to fit specific needs. For details, write SpecialMarkets@penguinrandomhouse.com.

Library of Congress Cataloging-in-Publication Data

Names: Light, Zuzka.
Title: 15 minutes to fit : the simple 30-day guide to total fitness, 15 minutes at a time / by Zuzka Light and Jeff O'Connell.
Other titles: Fifteen minutes to fit
Description: New York : AVERY an imprint of Penguin Random House, [2015]
Identifiers: LCCN 2015026720 | ISBN 9781583335826
Subjects: LCSH: Physical fitness.
Classification: LCC GV481 .L638 2015 | DDC 613.7—dc23
LC record available at http://lccn.loc.gov/2015026720

Printed in the United States of America

1 3 5 7 9 10 8 6 4 2

BOOK DESIGN BY LEE FUKUI AND MAUNA EICHNER

Dedicated to my followers around the world

Contents

Preface

Despite the balmy Mediterranean weather, sweat poured off my body—that's how hard I was training. Heaving with exhaustion, I tackled the final set of burpees. Don't let the cute name fool you: Burpees are a tough, wildly effective way to blast fat and build lean muscle.

The locals on Malta seemed perplexed by the sight of an eastern European woman in a sports bra with a firm stomach hopping up and down as though the rooftop—where we were filming this workout—were on fire, but I was doing exactly that. I'm sure these witnesses thought I was crazy.

From a standing position, I dropped into a squat and placed my palms on the ground. Without hesitating I kicked my legs back and assumed the top of a push-up position. I performed the push-up, and then, without hesitation, I drew my legs back into the low squat stance, glutes near the ground, before driving my body upward. I dropped into another rep and then another and another. I had no weights, no equipment, no gym, but I was cranking out reps of the most effective exercise that I think you can perform: Burpees work more than 200 muscles during each rep while leaving you gasping for additional oxygen after a set. This may exhaust you, but it helps you grow, and it also helps you feel alive.

My husband at that time, Freddy, recorded the entirety of this workout in Malta. We spent much of our tentative marriage traveling to far-flung locations and filming my daily workouts, posting them on YouTube and our website. The first of these

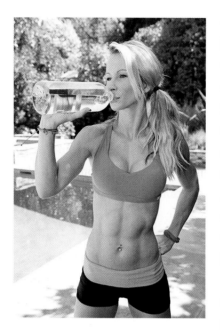

workouts was filmed in Prague, where I was born and raised. Then we moved to Canada, where he was raised. But that day's workout took place in Malta, where the low cost of living and balmy California-like weather helped us film outdoors. I could take off my sweats and train in my sports bra and shorts, showcasing my abs without freezing off my glutes. At that time, I was in my early twenties, and I didn't understand how these short workout videos we made would change my life for the better over the following years.

In early 2008, Freddy and I launched our fledgling business BodyRock.tv. We started small—when we launched the first website, I was working in a flower shop owned by my in-laws in Kingston, Ontario, Canada—but still, I was sure that people would like it. I knew it would take a while before the website started to make money, at least a year, but I knew it was going to work. BodyRock.tv started slowly, but then our YouTube channel started growing like crazy. With our short, intense, no-gym-required workouts, Freddy and I were on to a new workout style that people embraced in droves. It took only six months for us to reach one million views.

I based my workouts on moves I could perform anywhere because we couldn't afford gym memberships. Almost all of the workouts I found online were either bodybuilding style and directed toward men, or yoga-oriented for women. Neither of these suited my goals of burning body fat and adding lean muscle, so I invented my own training style, taking a few elements from an upstart movement called Cross-Fit, others from Tabata training, and adding my own unique twist to every influence I liked and thought would be effective.

Sure, some of my YouTube viewers were guys tuning in because they liked to watch a woman work out. But women constituted 90 percent of my audience. Despite our remote locations and low-tech approach to making fitness videos, my workout videos became a global fitness sensation. Millions of BodyRockers were doing my workouts every day and posting their fat-loss stories online. So I kept it up; I posted a video of my workouts each day and poured my heart, soul, and sweat out on-camera, making each workout more intense than every other at-home workout program. My fans loved the outdoor setting of the videos we shot in Malta, where we moved to from Canada. Malta helped us in other, unexpected ways. Uploading a video to the Web took six hours on this remote island. The longer the video, the longer it took us to upload it. To save uploading time, my workouts became shorter and more intense, until I distilled them to 15 minutes of fat-burning moves done in nonstop fashion. Rest came only after the workout ended.

I think part of my appeal was that I didn't bark orders or emphasize counts as some fitness personalities do. I didn't tell people what to do. I merely performed my workouts from start to finish, grunting and sweating along with viewers who were in it with me every rep of the way. There was a realness to these YouTube workouts that many at-home fitness programs don't provide.

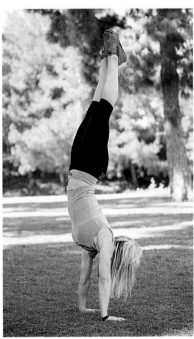

Canada and Malta seemed worlds apart, but no matter where we traveled, no matter how successful we became, I was always dogged by elements of my past and the threat of scandal. As a young woman living in Prague, I needed to make enough money to free myself from a troubled home life, which led me to make a regrettable decision: I posed nude for photos and video shoots. Like many young, vulnerable women, I found that this decision, once made, was nearly impossible to undo. In the Internet age, the consequences took on a life of their own. I worried that this would sabotage my newfound success once my followers learned about my past.

But something unexpected happened. When the full story of my earlier decisions began to trickle out in the comments sections of video postings, online forums, and other places, my popularity rose even faster. People now knew how much I had overcome. As my followers began to understand who I was and what I'd left behind, they seemed to appreciate me that much more. Most of them hadn't made the same mistakes I had made, but many of them had made their own mistakes. They identified with the struggles of a young woman trying to find success in our complicated world.

Huge social media followings and YouTube channels like mine drew the attention of large fitness companies. I found myself in Los Angeles meeting with Beachbody, Body by Jake, and other mainstream fitness brands because they had seen my YouTube workouts, and they were responding well to them. Something big was at hand.

My business and marriage were completely intertwined, however, and over the course of several years, that lack of separation doomed the marriage and drove a wedge between my husband and me. As our marriage dissolved, we became disgruntled and awkward business partners; and in the fallout, eventually I lost access to the website. The only thing I walked away with was my image. Rather than wallow in despair, I picked myself up and started over by launching a new website, ZuzkaLight.com. Today, I have surpassed my earlier success thanks to my current followers. Regardless of how you found me, I know that you're a woman or man taking control of your life by getting in better shape.

All my longtime followers know that I have helped them do this, and that's what I want to do for you. That's why I've written this book.

Introduction

I've often asked myself: Why me? With so many people posting so many workout videos online, why did so many viewers gravitate toward a young girl from the Czech Republic with an accent and no gym equipment? I've considered a number of theories, but I think so many people came to my YouTube videos for the workouts because they're highly effective. This book puts together a program based on these workouts in a novel way. These workouts do more than just burn fat and build muscle; they help unleash the super-fit person who lives inside each and every one of us. My followers learn they are able to perform harder workouts than they ever thought possible. This not only inspires confidence but teaches your muscles and body to learn what it's like to perform and train at peak levels.

Though at first it wasn't this clear to me, over time I came to realize that a real fitness philosophy lay behind my ideas and my approach. By using my inner turmoil to push myself harder during my workouts, I was tapping into the importance of high-intensity training. Science has now shown that intensity, along with consistency, is the key to workout success. That's true from both a performance and an aesthetic perspective.

Because YouTube is all about short videos, I was tapping into the power of short-burst workouts, which are both highly effective and compatible with a busy life like mine and, I imagine, yours. I had to come up with more and more high-intensity concepts that could be played over and over in a short-form format. Nobody wanted the half-hour blocks of workout shows that used to be shown on TV. Those shows had all vanished from the airwaves.

Because we didn't have much money and traveled around so much, weights and a gym were luxuries, not essentials. I crafted body weight workouts using the full body, which are now practiced and preached on mainstream websites and in magazines.

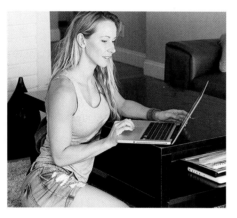

These are the principles I've built my brand around, and now I'm pleased to use them in my very first book. *15 Minutes to Fit* follows the same pattern as my videos. As you'll see in the pages to come, I provide a 30-day workout and nutrition plan that you can execute in a series of short-form set pieces that can be read and applied in 15 minutes, just like my YouTube workouts. In that sense, the book echoes my video workouts, but with a twist. Each 15-minute video workout is self-contained but ultimately is a limited fitness experience. Whereas the YouTube videos were individual workouts without any broader context, the book is a focused program that also encompasses nutrition. To that end, my book integrates multiple workouts, recipes, and motivational tips into a plan that can be followed from start to finish for awesome results.

The 15-minute limit applies to *everything* in this book. Everyone wants information fast and quick these days. Tweets cannot be longer than 140 characters. Vines can't exceed 6.5 seconds. Snapchats vanish nearly the instant they're viewed. And while *15 Minutes to Fit* gives you that same sense of immediacy by timing every element in the book, it will stay with you anywhere you go.

"Fifteen minutes to fit" may sound like some cheesy marketing slogan, but my program is based on science, and when you give it your all and push yourself to the limit each and every workout, as I do, you'll see incredible results. The workouts in *15 Minutes to Fit* consist of body weight exercises done in rapid-fire succession for as many rounds as possible until 15 challenging minutes of work have been completed. These short, high-intensity workouts jack up your heart rate and send your metabolic machinery into overdrive. They provide what repetitive crunches won't: visible abs, a round and tight butt, and toned arms. And, by the way, crunches will develop your abs but they won't make them visible—that's one of the big differences between this program and others. Having to regularly blast through existing fatigue thresholds builds power and stamina of the sort that also helps us be strong and capable in our everyday lives. You'll find that these workouts not only give you plenty of time for all other aspects of your life but also give you additional energy to accomplish more throughout your day.

I follow an innovative format that wraps cardio exercises around other moves. The body is constantly trying to adapt and, therefore, is continuously changing. The exercises by themselves are not complicated, but when they're arranged in this unique "wrapping" format, they challenge your mind and change your body. Throughout this book, the workouts keep evolving, with different workouts zeroing in on different problem areas, such as abs and butt.

My *15 Minutes to Fit* plan gives you what you need to take control of your body. You will shed pounds and build toned, sexy muscle without having to buy any equipment or even purchase a gym membership. I've been showcasing my workouts on YouTube and websites for nearly a decade now, and I've honed my approach over that time. I've taken all of that self-experimentation and written this fitness book, which takes my approach to a new level. I'm taking the guesswork out of getting ripped.

Every day for an entire month, you'll know exactly what to do, and you'll also receive a little pep talk from me. You'll be working out for 30 days straight, which may seem like a lot, but it's manageable. Because these workouts require only your body to perform and because they take only 15 minutes, you can work out every day. My program is not like traditional weight training, in which training days need to be separated by rest days. There's no need to be worried about overdoing it here.

For the workouts to create their magic, you also need to square away your diet. This book will help you in that regard because I provide detailed instructions in later chapters. The goal is for you to learn how to eat right naturally, without making it an obsession.

The workouts will give you a great-looking body and enhanced physical strength as well as inner calm. Challenging workouts are my form of daily meditation, as strange as that sounds. I've always had a hard time sitting still and meditating by just focusing on my breath, the way yogis teach. I can't fathom how people sit motionless thinking of nothing for 10 or 20 minutes at a time. My mind just won't settle down in that situation. But a funny thing happens during my short, intense workouts: I push all the negative energy out of me by tearing it up during my workout, and then I enjoy the relief that comes after the last rep. I'm so "in the moment" that nothing else occurs to me. That's the form of meditation I love, and that's why I can never give up on my fitness. It's as much mental as it is physical for me. These high-intensity workouts produce the high that comes with the endorphin release associated with being in the zone—let's call it the "Zuzka Zone." I'll show you how to get there throughout the book. I also love the bliss and calmness that come afterward. That's part of why I train.

I don't pretend my workouts are easy. Nor do I make them out to be a secret concoction made in some mysterious or magical exercise laboratory. What I do emphasize are efficiency and hard work. By hard work, I don't mean grueling, backbreaking routines, either. I mean effective, intelligent workout plans that offer visible results.

I train 15 minutes a day, but you may question whether that is realistic for you. Initially, if you can't sustain 15 minutes of high-intensity training, do it as long as possible, and then finish out your 15 minutes with easier work to encourage endurance. Eventually you will increase the amount of time you can train with high intensity. Let's say you're 35 pounds overweight. Chances are that you're not as fit as I am—not *yet*, anyway—and initially don't expect to exercise at the level of intensity that I now sustain for 15 minutes. After even a minute or two, you might be feeling a little winded. You may even feel a bit overwhelmed. That's fine. Do these workouts at your own level of "high" intensity, and you'll find you have more stamina with each new workout.

As a beginner, you have an advantage I no longer have. When you first begin working out and eating more healthfully, you may lose quite a bit of weight fairly quickly—more than I could lose even if I wanted to. Eventually, as you get lean and fit and have less fat to burn, the weight loss will slow, and you might find yourself thinking, "Wow, at first I lost weight really fast, but for some reason, I can't lose the last five pounds." I asked Ashley A. Herda, PhD, CSCS*D, a lecturer and academic program associate in the Department of Health, Sport, and Exercise Sciences at the University of Kansas (Edwards), why pretty much everyone eventually experiences a slowdown in their progress. "Early on, a lot of the weight lost is going to come from water loss and some fat loss," she said. "If you are losing weight at first but then the loss is slowing down, you may actually be gaining muscle while losing fat. A study conducted at Syracuse University reported that obese women actually burned *more* fat during an exercise bout than their nonobese counterparts. The authors concluded that the reduction in fat stores resulted in less fat being available to use as energy."

In other words, the more fat you lose, the less fat you burn.

So don't get discouraged when the weight loss slows. On this plan, you'll constantly adjust your training and diet to reflect that your body is becoming leaner, stronger, more efficient. It takes time. Part of that adaptation is being able to work a lot harder during those 15 minutes than you could previously. "As your training progresses," says Dr. Herda, "your body becomes a more efficient machine. Every movement is more coordinated by the working muscles, where early on these same muscles were working against one another—a sort of safety mechanism to protect your body from injury. Initially, you would recruit only large muscle groups to complete a movement, but eventually you'll also call upon smaller muscles you never knew you had to help out with the more complex movements. Fifteen minutes becomes less of a struggle and way more enjoyable, knowing you are benefiting from every single movement."

The biggest motivation for me at this moment is to create the best workouts I can for people who want to be fitter. I want to do these workouts myself so other people can achieve the level of fitness they want and be happy with how they feel and look. I created this book so that readers will be able to take the philosophy everywhere they go. Armed with these words and images, you'll be able to succeed without having to rely on anyone or anything else. I'm confident that the 30-day plan in this book works because it worked for me and, more important, because this style of training has worked for thousands of women and men who have followed me for nearly a decade.

15

Minutes
to FIT

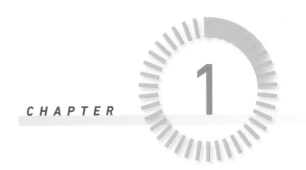

The Spark

Nearly every single fitness magazine and product on the market catches our eye with toned abs or a tight butt, laced together with promises on how to achieve such perfection. We look at these images with envy, thinking that these people walk around chiseled 24/7, 365. The magazines make a point *not* to explain that the image was taken on the day that person was in the best shape of her life, with perfect lighting, and that afterward that image may have been edited to remove any lingering imperfections. It creates an urge to want to have the same body, and the willingness to do whatever it takes sets in. It's a compelling pitch because we all want a cute butt and small-size jeans. So we gaze at those images, look at ourselves in the mirror, and then start our journey of transforming our body.

This *external motivation* starts millions on the fitness path, but for the vast majority of those individuals, this path ends in a dead end. The needle on the scale doesn't move fast enough, that miraculous body doesn't appear overnight, and they give up. Oftentimes these individuals try and try again, until they finally give up for good. Their mind didn't fully buy into what their body tried, which happens all too often and *not* just where working out is concerned.

I believe these people were doomed to fail from the get-go because they were too hung up on appearances, the models' and their own. What they needed was *internal motivation*, the sort that comes from within and is validated by changes that don't always show up in the mirror—changes like a nice glow, more energy, more strength, and a heightened sense of confidence. I have experienced all those benefits firsthand, and it's why fitness infuses every part of my life and being. Because those benefits propel me to train every day, I now enjoy a shapely butt, a defined midsection, a nice pair of legs that fit comfortably in skinny jeans. Those visuals, however, are a bonus. At this point I'm more addicted to the way my workouts make me feel than I am to the way they make me look. I'm compelled to do them. You couldn't stop me from working out if you tried.

Exercise offers many immediate benefits, not just physical but mental as well. Training the way I do helps me fight stress and anxiety. I don't know one person who walks out of a gym, cardio class, or yoga studio after a good workout feeling unhappy or stressed. Tired, maybe, but the sort of tired that accompanies a job well done. Exercise helps send your troubles packing, replacing them with inner calm.

Fitness also offers tremendous long-term benefits. It helps with weight management. It keeps you flexible and graceful. It keeps your heart strong and healthy. It helps keeps your bones strong. One of the reasons I work out is that I want to be healthy and strong in the future if and when I have children.

Exercise: The Real Fountain of Youth

Moderate physical activity decreases the risk of cardiovascular disease, stroke, and mortality from all causes, even if the activity starts later in life. A study conducted in Canada, which reported similar findings as the Harvard Alumni Health Study in 1995, recorded the physical activity of 14,365 men and women across their life-span and reported that the more one exercises, the greater one's life expectancy. Even if they were exercising at only low intensities, their all-cause mortality risk was reduced.

Too often people don't stick with it long enough to see physical results. That part of the equation takes patience, and patience is something few maintain while trying to achieve a big goal, especially when it involves physical changes. It is almost as though if physical changes haven't appeared in 20 minutes or less, we assume nothing happened and therefore exercise is no longer worth the effort. However, lack of quick physical changes is not the only cause of failure. Of-

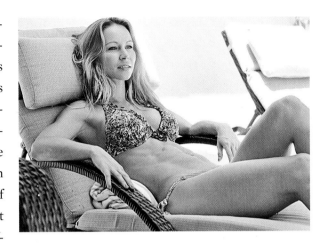

ten, the workout plans these people follow are unnecessarily long and dull, and people lose patience with that aspect of fitness too. If they're working with a personal trainer, they might come to view that person as Satan himself. They dread their workouts and drag themselves through what feels like 60 to 90 minutes of sheer misery. And we wonder why so many people quit.

Finding the Right Reason

If you've hated exercising in the past, you're not alone. In May 2014, I sat in the audience at the Saban Theater in Beverly Hills, watching Jillian Michaels onstage. She's known across the world for her tenure as one of the tough-love trainers on *The Biggest Loser*, the beloved and inspirational NBC-TV show. This appearance was part of her "Maximize Your Life" tour, and her lecture—that's the best way I can describe it—was entertaining and eye opening. It reminded me of the *An Inconvenient Truth* movement, only rather than addressing climate change, Jillian was talking about the declining state of public health in the United States. Sometimes people refuse to accept the evidence right in front of their face, because it has accumulated slowly enough that the changes are imperceptible. She was explaining what each of us could do to make a difference.

I watched this fitness icon share her wisdom and offer advice on how to diet, exercise, and stay fit. Beyond sets, reps, and calories, she talked about the intangibles that help determine whether someone transforms her body or ends up planted on the sofa eating a bag of Doritos. At one point, this woman whom I have admired for years asked the audience a question: "Who among you actually enjoys working out?" There were three hundred people in the audience, but only three raised their hands.

You may be surprised that so few people felt that way, but I wasn't. I know, based on my own experience with training others, that many people dislike working out. Even Jillian Michaels, of all people, admitted that she dislikes it. "Well, great," you could almost hear people thinking. "If Jillian Michaels can't stand working out, for crying out loud, what hope do I have?" And yet, nearly every day of her adult life, Jillian puts amazing effort into something she says she dislikes, because it gives her the body and life she wants.

Making Fitness Fun

I was one of three people in attendance who raised a hand in response to Jillian Michaels's question. You could say I'm one of those few weirdos who actually enjoys physical exercise, but that's only scratching the surface. I've found a fitness formula that turns working out from drudgery into fun, so that the workouts themselves are a form of intrinsic motivation. The program isn't overwhelming, so you don't give up before those visible results start appearing.

My workouts are also incredibly efficient, producing the results I want in the time I have, and the resulting benefits provide extrinsic motivation. Sure, there are days when I have a hard time getting my butt up off the couch—or even squeezing a workout between "more important" tasks, like most people do. However, I have come up with enough reasons to overcome scheduling excuses and step out of my own comfort zone. One reason is that I'm going to be training for only 15 minutes, not 90 minutes. Even if I'm having an off day, as long as I dive in and start training, I know I will finish strong and the rest of my goals for that day won't suffer.

Internal Motivation

When it comes to fitness, it has to be about the payoff of the "high" that comes from training. That is what leads to great physical and performance results. Just trying to avoid feeling fat or unfit isn't enough. You have to derive pleasure from the workouts you perform and the foods you eat. The pleasure can be external, as per Jillian Michaels, or it can be internal, as it is with me.

I avoid exercise boredom by keeping my workouts short and by structuring them as challenges or competitions. Most of us love to compete or at least compare our results to others. I ask you to perform my workouts as fast as possible within the allotted 15 minutes. It's about what you accomplish in that time frame. I ask you to post your score and compare yours with that of others. Once you start doing that, you'll get pumped. You'll start thinking, "Oh, I can compete now, and I want to do better and really push myself." I've learned that this really helps keep people motivated.

ZGYM, the subscription section of my website, is where the workouts become motivating: when the community gets together and everyone is focused on their performance and beating each other's scores or being able to do certain new

> *It is clear that we must trust what is difficult.*
> —RAINER MARIA RILKE

exercises. I can't tell you how many times I've heard things like "I've never tried this exercise before, and I'm going to kill it," or similar sentiments. That motivates me to keep creating new exercises and combining them into new workouts. People find it motivating and their motivation is contagious, and that provides a feedback loop of good vibes and achievement.

Maybe you've struggled with workout motivation, and if you'd been in the audience watching Jillian Michaels, you wouldn't have raised your hand when she asked if you like to work out. Luckily, you've come to the right place. I'm going to give you a guide not only about how to work out and get results but also how to enjoy it. Fitness, motivation, desire, compulsion, and the workout high are one and the same in my world.

Every human was born to exert his or her body; there's a reason we have those two limbs attached to our hips and two to our shoulders. We were made to move, not sit around on our butts all day. In my experience, the reason people dread going to the gym is that their gym routines have become boring. We weren't made to pound the treadmill mindlessly for an hour and a half, which must be why many gyms hang TV screens in the cardio area. They might as well hang a sign that says: "You're going to be really freaking bored doing this, so here, watch this."

External Motivation

Something else keeps people motivated: physical results! In turn, results lead to positive reinforcement. You start working out. Maybe you're not always enjoying it, but then suddenly people start looking at you in a different light. Others seem to find you more attractive. You catch your significant other looking at you in a new light, and the realization sends a shiver down your spine. That's a catalyst to continue upping your game.

This type of motivation is powerful, but the key to success on my plan or any plan is to couple this with internal motivation. It's impossible to be self-sufficient if you constantly rely on input from others. You never know when external motivation will be unavailable, and you also become susceptible to negative feedback. When you believe in what you're doing, the external input might give you a nice boost when it's positive, but it won't bring you down when it's negative.

Our external motivation needs to change over the years because we change. When I started out in fitness, my motivation was seeing fit people with beautiful bodies. I wanted to look that good. Today that no longer cuts it for me. I need more. I need to see somebody who embodies dedication by playing a sport at a high level, for example. When I see people playing tennis or skiing, I'm excited and hence motivated by a skill that was built off of being fit. I wrote earlier about those who don't heed the call when confronted with what others would see as a catalyst. Still others heed the call, only to attempt a transformation and fail. Like a spark that doesn't light a fire, their effort fizzles.

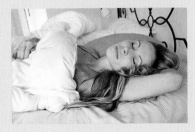
Catching the Fitness Bug

When it comes to fitness, we all have to start somewhere. If I had to trace my love affair with fitness back to one moment, it was during the summer of 1997, when I was a 15-year-old girl living in the Czech Republic. I was born and raised in the capital city of Prague. It's one of Europe's great cities, steeped in history and teeming with beautiful architecture and people. One day I went with a group of friends to a showing of *G.I. Jane*, a movie starring Demi Moore. We wanted to kill some time and escape the outside world for a couple hours.

Once Demi Moore appeared on screen as Lieutenant Jordan O'Neill, I was transfixed. This character personified beauty, strength, and power. Her physique, short hair, and attitude symbolized her ability to kick ass, and this sent my imagination into overdrive. As the movie continued, I loved seeing her become super-strong and compete with the guys. By the time my friends and I left the theater, I wanted to *become* Lieutenant Jordan O'Neill, even if I didn't know if I could attain that status. But that movie gave me two things I didn't have when I entered the theater: a goal and a role model.

For several weeks after seeing *G.I. Jane*, I couldn't get that movie out of my head. I knew I needed to work out because it was clear that physical fitness was why Demi Moore's character had so much inner strength. If I wanted to be like her, I knew I needed to do what she'd done to get that way. I needed to train.

To do that, I knew I needed to join a gym. The only one I knew of was in the basement under a complex of doctors' offices in Prague. It was called Fitness Troja. This was the same complex where I went for so many of my doctor appointments as a child. Now I was there for another reason, and I found myself walking down a long, dark hallway, which led to a door that led into the gym. It felt strange to be in the unfamiliar basement of a building I thought I knew so well. The closer I got, the more I could smell the musty scent of a basement full of men. From outside I could hear noises within, grunts and yells and clanking metal. I was scared even to open the door, and several times I turned to leave. But I really wanted to work out. So I waited at the door for 10 minutes before deciding to open it.

I entered a very plain, gray, rough-around-the-edges kind of place. I knew every doctor and all the nurses in the building, but here I felt completely alien and alone. Two things hit me immediately. First, I was the youngest person in the room. Second, there was only one other woman working out. She worked there, as it turned out, and her body looked amazing, even though she looked 10 years older than I was. She reminded me of Xena, the heroine of a television series about a warrior princess— muscular but in an attractive way.

I never actually talked to "Xena" or any of her friends whom I would see later at the gym. I was too shy. At first, I didn't know how to exercise like she did. In fact, I was totally clueless about working out. I asked a guy who worked there for help, and he was so intimidating I thought he was being mean to me at first. He was talking to me as if I were just another gym dude. He didn't offer gentle encouragement; he just set me on the machine and barked in a gruff voice, "This is what you do!"

His name was Standa, and he turned out to be a really cool guy who was always trying his best to make a living with this little gym to support his family. He would always hang out with a few guys who worked out at the gym every day. They used to tease me when I was a teenager, but we all became good friends over the years, encountering each other at the gym and around the neighborhood. Few girls would show up at his gym to work out, but I didn't mind. I was always very focused on my training whenever I went to the gym—even though I had no idea what I was doing.

Eventually, Standa let me be the instructor for Spinning classes in his gym because he had enrolled more female members and they all expressed interest in taking group classes. He had only eight bikes, so I could brag that my classes were always full. Fitness was addictive. If I had nothing else to do, I would just go to the gym for a workout. Without a doubt, I was hooked.

The beginning of my transition to at-home training came when I bought a videocassette of *The Next Challenge Workout* with Cindy Crawford. I got so hooked that I was doing it almost every day. I remember it being really hard and having to pause the video every 10 minutes. I couldn't understand how it was possible that she didn't even break a sweat! At that point I had access to only one decent TV channel and no Internet connection. I had no idea how shooting a video actually worked.

Working out with Cindy Crawford helped me to see my abs for the very first time. It was just a faint outline, but it made me happy and even more motivated. I dreamed about what it would be like having my own DVD and being able to shoot in some beautiful location. If someone told me that would in fact be my job one day, I never would have believed it.

When Motivation Strikes

Motivation is a miraculous concept, and we all need that first spark to illuminate the darkness, if only for a split second. However, that spark, while essential, is not enough, largely because it's elusive and unreliable. I didn't enter the movie theater in Prague that day expecting any great awakening. I didn't even know that I was sleepwalking through my life and that I needed awakening. I was killing a few hours with my friends. The lightbulb turned on in my head without warning, and the woman who exited from that theater when the house lights came on was different from the one who had entered it.

Perhaps you've had random encounters or experiences that fired you up about some new hobby or undertaking. Maybe something happened deep inside when you least expected it, and afterward your life was no longer the same. I'll bet that your life has included several such pivot points.

> *Life is really simple, but we insist on making it complicated.*
> —CONFUCIUS

Those moments are exceptional. More often, we search, usually in vain, for motivation. We scroll through our Facebook and Twitter feeds to see if something creates enough of a spark to propel us off the couch and send us to the gym. We thumb through fitness magazines in the supermarket checkout line when a fit body or clever cover line catches our eye. We see a colleague at work who has successfully transformed and ask her for her secret, in hopes that we too can shape up. We scan our iPod for a track that might fire us up. We hold up an old pair of jeans, thinking, "God, I'd *love* to fit in these again."

We shouldn't be constantly hunting for external motivation, nor do we necessarily need to have it all the time. This hunt for motivation is actually more like a fishing expedition. You cast your line and hope something bites, unsure if anything will. Who knows? You won't always find motivation and hence can't rely on it. You may think you do, only you don't. You might leave the theater, or wherever your epiphany happened, feeling pumped up, fired up, and ready to take on the world like I did that day in Prague. However, when you awaken the next morning, it's raining outside . . . or you have a headache . . . or your period is particularly bad. Those are hypothetical, but any sort of life event can short-circuit your motivation. Don't get me wrong, motivation is great and can excite you about working out. However, it's hit or miss. Therefore it can't be counted on to sustain a lasting transformation.

One of my followers, who posts on my website as Self-Care Diva, sums it up perfectly:

> We grudgingly spend time going to the bank or the grocery store or dropping kids off at school, and we don't expect ourselves to be super-excited about those things. Health and fitness are really difficult to prioritize when the advertising messages are all about making life "simpler" with processed foods and pills to take in place of exercise; billboards featuring

beautiful, fit-looking individuals drinking Cokes or eating Chicken McNuggets. We are swimming upstream against these messages, so *of course* motivation will fluctuate. I try to replace the word *motivation* with *persistence*. It validates that there is an actual struggle and that it *is* hard to stay on track sometimes. The idea is to commit and persist.

There's a meme I've seen on social media that I love. It's a drawing of a woman jumping rope, and the caption says, "What am I training for? Life, motherfucker!" Success in fitness and life requires hard work, discipline, and occasionally the willingness to do boring stuff. Diet and exercise are not always fun or exciting. Sometimes it seems like a chore when we're tired and our bodies crave comfort. While it's necessary to reward ourselves from time to time by indulging here and there, it's important to view diet and exercise as a challenge that is constantly contributing to our growth as human beings. Competitive athletes often talk about mind-set being a key to their success. Focus on the challenge of fitness and how it's positively affecting your life with each passing day. Remember, well-being is earned, not given.

Finding a Catalyst

Often what drives people to take the plunge is a sense of dissatisfaction or unrest, perhaps even shame. Something about their life feels wrong, and it occurs to them that they can fix it in the gym. And I believe this is true. I believe the word *bodybuilding* is misleading, in fact; for many people, the gym is more of a repair shop for poor self-esteem, subpar health, and other issues. Before people can build themselves, they must put themselves back together mentally, physically, and emotionally. For many people, their exercise is an exercise in self-image building.

The specifics are unique for everyone, although certain themes recur in many transformation stories. Maybe it's seeing a friend get in shape and wanting that for yourself. Maybe it's a health scare or a moment of shame. Maybe it's an intervention from friends, family members, or both, challenging you to get your act together. It could even be a fictitious character who inspires you, like Lieutenant Jordan O'Neill in my case. The spark is different for each of us.

Mind over Body

To avoid procrastination, I imagine how I'll feel 15 to 20 minutes from now, *after* my workout: out of breath, soaked in sweat, happy and proud that I completed my workout. I know how much more energized I'll feel after my workout, and I love that state of mind. It takes me only a minute to get in the mood. Then I just have to start, and once I start, I can't stop.

You can also imagine yourself 20 minutes from now if you choose not to do your workout. What exactly is going to change? Nothing. Your mood and energy are going to be the same, and you'll most likely feel bad that you just gave up on yourself. Doing this simple mind game really does help me stop procrastinating and do my workout. Besides that, I like to remind myself that all I need is 15 minutes.

People receive wake-up calls all the time, but many of them turn a deaf ear to their own call. Taking the initiative to pick up this book tells me that you heard the call and you want to act on it. To do so successfully means reaching a point where working out and eating nutritious foods become second nature, to where they become daily habits much like brushing your teeth, going to bed at night, or driving to work. You don't even think twice about doing these activities, and your fitness and nutrition programs will become automatic too.

I started off training in a gym, but eventually I began working out at home. I wanted to feel that, wherever I might go, even if I didn't have access to the Internet, even if I couldn't talk to anyone about fitness, even if there were no gym, I could stay in shape. I wanted to be strong and independent. As I write this paragraph, I haven't stepped in a gym in seven years. And I don't miss it *at all*. But the point is that I continued to follow my fitness regimen regardless of where I was or what I was doing. No gym was no excuse. I could have been on an island or at the North Pole, and I still would have trained because I was motivated, and that made all the difference in the world.

Fitness isn't complicated. It's actually quite simple, but simple does not in any way mean *easy*. There shouldn't be a whole lot of mystery or head scratching when you're getting in shape. Instead, there should be a lot of sweat and a fair amount of discipline in the kitchen and elsewhere. Those of you who have already experienced my workouts on YouTube or ZuzkaLight.com know this to be true. There are no magic

> *Simplicity is the ultimate sophistication.*
> —LEONARDO DA VINCI

potions, contraptions, or secret techniques to transforming your body by gaining muscle and losing fat. There is only one real solution: consistent effort. If you're just starting with me, know that you have the strength and willpower within you to transform yourself inside and out with simplicity and consistency. It's there, I promise!

NEVER GIVE UP PROFILE
Mary Scott

I've been fascinated with bicycles since childhood. I viewed my bike not just as a form of transportation but also an instrument of freedom. Eventually I began competing in local and regional races and did well in my category. Like many young people, I dreamed of being either an Olympic or a professional athlete—maybe even both! However, my practical side won out, and I chose to attend college instead. Yet the cycling bug never left me. For the next 10 years, I entered races in both road and cross-country cycling.

One day I crashed my bike and shattered my arm, which required multiple surgeries. Realizing that competitive cycling was no longer an option, I began looking for a new form of exercise. I needed to be able to exercise on my timetable, within a very limited amount of time, regardless of the hour of day. I chose to explore body weight exercises, and while researching this topic, I discovered Zuzka Light. I loved that the exercises she demonstrates require a minimum investment in equipment and that everything can be completed at home and on my schedule. *(continues)*

I'm challenged by any exercise that requires placing heavy forces on one arm or requires wrist flexion—for example, a one-arm push-up! These moves test my weakness and make me stronger in the process. The repertoire of routines Zuzka has published pushes me to try exercises that both challenge me and keep me interested. I may have lost my love for cycling—but I found a new love in body weight circuit training!

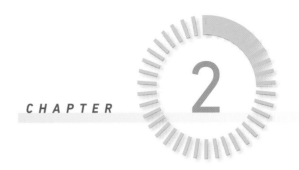

CHAPTER 2

The Steps to Achievement

O nce you pinpoint your motivation—whether it's to have fun with exercise again, to fit back into a specific pair of jeans, or whatever it is—it's time to set goals for yourself. Most people set goals all the time but don't achieve them. It takes a spark of inspiration—as I discussed in Chapter 1—and a whole lot of discipline.

Goals are about more than just losing that muffin top. They can reflect what you want to achieve in your noon workout (short term) or where you want to be ten years from now (long term). Ideally, your short-term goals feed into the long-term goals to such a degree that success in the long-term goals takes on an air of inevitability. If you consistently meet your goal of crushing that noon workout, you stand a very good chance of being where you want to be body-wise in ten years. Obviously the reverse is true as well: If you're not hitting those daily marks, you're going to be *way* off course in a decade.

One of my goals is for you to read this book and begin following my 30-day workout plan. But before I reach *my* goal, I want to help you reach *yours*.

Setting Good Goals

When setting a goal, it's not enough to just say, "I want to be leaner and drop a few pounds," or "I really want to get rid of the muffin top before my wedding." Those are desires, not goals. They're not specific enough, and as a result, they seldom lead to success. That desire is seldom fulfilled. It remains wishful thinking.

If you want to lose weight and have more muscle tone, for example, formulate an idea of *specifically* how much weight you want to lose and what body fat percentage you hope to achieve. Good goals are three things: (1) specific, (2) measurable, and (3) realistic. Better to say, "My goal is to lose 20 pounds before Christmas Day [or by my wedding on such-and-such day]." Twenty pounds is a specific number, and the idea of losing that weight by Christmas is measurable. Assuming you're far enough removed from Christmas, this goal is realistic too.

Worthwhile goals tend to be emotionally charged so that they always motivate you to keep going and not give up. If your goal has Christmas as its end date, it's easy to get super excited about that too, in part because your entire family will see your achievement—assuming you spend the holidays with them. That excitement is a very important part of the success equation, and that's why your goal needs to be emotionally charged. A high school reunion offers the same kind of charge. Maybe you were overweight in high school and bullied as a result. Imagine the satisfaction you would get from going to that event looking like a million bucks!

For many of you, the most important long-term goal will be a lower body weight. In establishing this goal, make your "dream weight" healthy and proportionate to your height. If you are a woman and the same height as I am, five foot five, your ideal body weight falls somewhere between 113 and 138 pounds. That's a healthy range, which is the most important thing. As I write this, I weigh 122 pounds. If I wanted to be thinner, I could still drop nine pounds without becoming underweight. It isn't healthy to lose any more than that, though. So having this knowledge is important for avoiding unhealthy weight loss.

Take some time and think about your long-term goals. Where do you want to be in three months? In a year? In five years? In ten years? Write these goals down—that very act can help bring clarity to your thought process. There's a reason people keep diaries; it helps them take inventory of what's happening in their life. Well, I want you to write about the future, and in a way that can come true and not be science fiction.

One thing I don't want you to do is aim low in your ambitions, whether it be in the gym or in life. Guys are expected to dream big and forge an interesting and lucrative career. If they don't, people will call them slackers. As for women, too often we are discouraged from dreaming big. We're supposed to marry the man of our dreams, have babies, serve our husband, and dote on our kids, with little concern for carving our own path through life. I'm all about empowering women and girls to think big. You can do whatever you want in life, and your success and happiness don't hinge on anyone else. Unfortunately, many women are still not empowered. In many places around the world, women lack basic human dignity. They are denied simple rights such as the right to work, to drive, and to vote. They are persecuted if they even express the desire to challenge the status quo. I want you to aim high and bust out of the traps women get sucked into.

> *The strongest of all warriors are these two: Time and Patience.*
>
> —LEO TOLSTOY

Achieving Your Goals

Once your goals are not only set but also written down, you need to figure out how to achieve them. I want you to reverse-engineer your actions from those ultimate goals by setting small daily goals that are essentially stepping-stones bringing you closer to your long-term goals. Saying that you want to lose 10 pounds in three months means nothing until you write down what it will take to get there. If you focus too much on large goals and not the specific steps that take you there, it's easy to become overwhelmed and frustrated. If mountain climbers focus on the size of the mountain rather than the very next step in front of them, they'll never reach the top, and they might even get injured during their ascent.

Let's say that today is September 9 and you want to lose 20 pounds before Christmas Day. You have 107 days, or 15 weeks, to realize your dream. You need to craft a plan consisting of smaller goals. Those daily goals are your "behavior goals," and they represent a series of small ongoing commitments. You need to write them down just like you did your long-term goal. For example:

1. I commit to working out five times a week and then to do some fun activity that at least will get me moving on the other days too.

2. I commit to eating only the number of calories that I need to achieve my ultimate goal. (See the chart on page 85 for how to determine your necessary caloric intake.)

3. I commit to eating lean protein, veggies and/or fruit, and healthy fats with every meal.

4. I commit to eating added sugar and/or starchy carbs only within the window that ends two hours after my workout.

5. I commit to weighing myself each week and adjusting my caloric intake accordingly. (You don't want to eat the same amount of food that you were eating when you were 10 pounds heavier, so it's a good idea to do this every week.)

From there, take it day by day—and don't even worry about 20 pounds or Christmas Day, both of which could feel overwhelming. Each morning, commit to doing your workout or your other activity if it's an active rest day. Wake up with a small goal, nail it, and then go to sleep feeling successful and accomplished. The same thing applies with your diet. Always wake up thinking, *Today will be a successful day.* That way you can celebrate each day as a small victory. You may not be able to control your fat cells and your metabolic rate, but you can control the actions you take that lead to a lean and athletic body.

You also need to be flexible. Things won't always go your way. I guarantee it. When that happens, will you adapt and keep going, or will you fold up your tent and go home? If you're falling behind on a certain timeline, figure out if you can make up the difference later on. Maybe you went through a really tough stretch at work and missed some of your workouts as a result. Accept that reality and figure out how you can get back on track. Later, you might encounter a stretch where work is less demanding than usual, in which case you devote even more time to fitness. Things often even out in the end, but you won't know that unless you ride out those rough stretches.

See, goals of any duration take patience, especially when they are fitness goals. Nothing is more personal than our own body, so when it's not where we want it to be, we want to change it overnight. The fact that there are huge industries built around plastic surgeries, liposuction, fad diets, anabolic steroids, and weight loss pills speaks to this impulse. So many of these products and services prey on people's weaknesses and insecurities.

The approach I advocate takes time, energy, and hard work. I pride myself on the efficiency of my workouts and cooking, but while I don't waste time, there is work that needs to be done and exertion that must be put forth. Watch my videos—I *sweat*—and you'll understand what I'm saying. There's no getting around that basic truth. Fitness and well-being can feel like hard work because *they are* hard work. More often than

not, the things in life that help us grow and prosper are the most difficult. Eating an entire bag of chips while watching TV for five hours is easy. Sweating it out at the ZGYM, followed by preparing a healthy meal, is not so easy, but it is infinitely more rewarding for your body *and* your mind. That's one of the great things about fitness too. When you look fit and you're in great shape, people know you earned it.

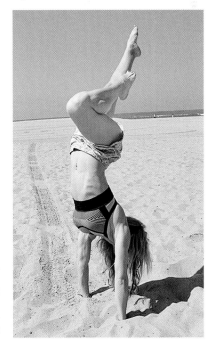

When we talk about fitness and well-being, it's not just about breaking a sweat, looking good, and eating your vegetables, though. Not that those things aren't important; they are hugely important. But fitness is more about redirecting the course of your life toward a healthier, infinitely more satisfying sense of *who you are.* This, of course, is no easy task. It not only requires diligence and hard work but also requires patience. Patience goes hand in hand with consistency. Slow and steady does, in fact, win the race. Often people give up, not because the challenge of fitness proves too difficult but because they lack patience and consistency.

My back became a big issue as recently as 2014. I felt horrible pain there. I could literally touch the disc that was bulging in my lumbar spine, and this caused shooting pain down my right leg, even though the disc was bulging toward the left. It was awful. I thought, "What am I going to do now?" And, of course, being a modern human being, I did an online search to find out what was going to happen to me. I thought, "I will have to have an operation, my body will never be the same, my career is over," and so forth.

So I went to a physiotherapist for an examination. He thought that I had a herniated disc, referring to the little "shock absorber" we all have in between our vertebrae. These discs allow our spine to bend and twist while remaining stable. The physiotherapist was concerned enough that he referred me to a spine doctor. The doctor wanted to operate, but I wasn't ready to go under the knife.

In the meantime, I tried all sorts of things, like acupuncture, but nothing seemed to help. I was popping eight ibuprofen pills a day. I was in horrible pain. I would take those medications right before we filmed my daily workout, just so I could survive them. Once the shoot was a wrap, pain would return for the rest of the day. Almost in desperation, I purchased a book called *Pain Free*, by Pete Egoscue and Roger Gittines. The authors argued that many disc problems of the sort I experienced can be treated through exercise rather than surgery. Your bones will do what your muscles tell them to do, they contend. Therefore our muscles can pull our bones into correct alignment. But when our muscles are too weak or too tight, bad things happen.

The Egoscue Method, as it's known, isn't intended as a quick fix. Healing my back would take patience, I read, and I accepted that reality. I started doing the exercises daily. At first I needed to do the exercises hourly to remain pain-free without taking pills, but then I had to do the exercises every four hours, and so on. Finally, I could do the exercises once a day. In one month, my spine was pain free, just like the title of that book. Just as an aside, I was so impressed with the results that I decided to study the Egoscue Method and receive my certification in it so that I can help people with problems like the one I experienced. It's the kind of technique I like: It empowers people. Once you give them the lessons, they can keep themselves healthy rather than relying on others for help. I'm a huge believer in self-sufficiency and independence.

Patience is often held up as a virtue but practicing it is another matter, unless you happen to be the Dalai Lama. More likely you can identify with one of my followers, Mélissa Bourbonnais, when she says: "I'm *so* impatient. I want everything immediately. The same holds true for me when it comes to my own health and fitness. I tried many diets and that led to a yoyo effect of gaining weight, losing it, gaining it back, and so forth. Two years ago I finally learned from my mistakes and developed self-control. Since that time, I've lost weight the healthiest way possible, through exercise and healthy diet. It takes time, but I've seen big changes. Now living in a healthy way has become a habit!"

> *You wait and watch and work: you don't give up.*
> —ANNE LAMOTT

Being patient may seem like a yawn-inducing chore. We want what we want and we want it now, and there's no point twiddling our thumbs, right? Wrong. Patience can be one of our greatest strengths. Patience allows us to steadily build our strength and stamina; to shed unwanted pounds in a healthy manner; and to endure, even thrive, during our hardest days or weeks of workouts. Patience gets us through our most difficult times in life and nurtures unforeseen strength and growth that might never have come about had we settled for a shortcut. We need to be patient whether we like it or not.

Patience is really about staying in the moment and not looking too far ahead, even though your goals have been set. To reach them requires focusing on one workout at a time, one meal at a time, one decision at a time, and so forth. It means keeping your eyes on the prize and not becoming distracted by the past.

Cut Yourself Some Slack

If for whatever reason you don't meet the goals you set for yourself, despite your best efforts, don't beat yourself up over it. One of my followers, Leigh Cooper, wrote to me to share her experience: "I checked my weight this morning to discover it hasn't budged in a week. I've worked out steadily, eaten great, and avoided alcohol for three weeks and my weight hasn't moved in seven days. I gave serious thought to spending the day binging on junk and feeling sorry for myself."

Sound familiar? I think we've all been there before.

Leigh continued: "But then I said no. Three weeks isn't nearly long enough. I've only just begun. And I'm not after a number here. I'm after a lifestyle. So here I am planning today's workout."

It's human nature to grow frustrated when goals are not met. This is particularly true when it comes to fitness. You may have a specific weight loss goal in mind, or maybe you're trying to master a difficult move like the pistol squat. Maybe you put in a fair amount of work, only to find your goal still out of reach. Instead of getting upset or frustrated, reward yourself for your hard work. You put in the time and the effort, and that's a worthy accomplishment in and of itself. More often than not, most good things in life take a little longer than expected. Set goals, but don't get bent out of shape when things don't go as planned. Adapt, move forward, and continue to work hard. You'll be surprised how effective and productive this approach can be.

NEVER GIVE UP PROFILE
Tanya Deckard

I'm 33 years old, married, and a Navy veteran. My husband is 34 years old and had been in pretty good shape when he was young. Unfortunately, once he got out of the Navy, he really let himself go. He wasn't very health conscious until early 2012, when he was diagnosed with a rare form of tongue cancer. The affected area was small, but the treatment involved removing all of his teeth as well as almost three-quarters of his tongue.

By the end of 10 weeks of radiation and chemo, this five-foot-eleven-inch man had dropped almost 80 pounds, to 142, and was still eating through a feeding tube. Because he was having a hard time putting on any weight after his recovery, he decided to hit the gym, where he gained 30 pounds in six months. For the first time in almost ten years, Josh was in better shape than I was, so that's when my fitness goals required a lifestyle change for me.

My husband challenged me to join him in doing the 2014 Tough Mudder event in Houston to celebrate his two-year anniversary of being cancer-free. He said that was what he wanted for his birthday. I really wanted to do it, so I knew I needed a serious game plan. I began bouncing around the Internet looking for workout plans and routines to help me on my quest. I found Zuzka after trying a few other programs. For the first time, I was beginning to see the results I wanted!

Cancer didn't beat my husband and me—we beat cancer! It took a positive attitude and dedication to our lifestyle change. Watching your loved one go through such a traumatic event and come out on top is truly remarkable and inspirational. I know that sometimes my husband would stop and watch me doing Z's workouts, and it motivated *him* to keep pushing. With time at the gym and eating healthy, Josh and I, along with three of our friends, completed this year's Tough Mudder event!

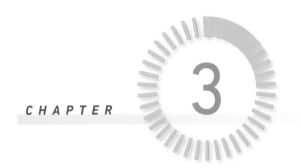

The Power of Habit, the Need for Consistency

You might find it hard to believe now, but when I was 20 years old, I was a chain smoker. I relied on cigarettes to calm my nerves during times of stress and to make me feel more comfortable in social situations.

Ironically, growing up in Prague, I *hated* being around smokers. My mother would smoke all day long, starting with her morning coffee. We lived in a small apartment, which meant there was no escaping it; curtains that used to be white turned yellow. My brother developed asthma and I believe it was a result of constant exposure to secondhand smoke. I would get so mad at my mom that I'd say, "Why do you smoke around us? Why do you need to smoke at home? You're going to get sick!"

No matter what I said, no matter how hard I implored her to stop, she wouldn't.

I moved out of my mother's home when I was 18, and when I was 20, *I* started smoking. I was around friends who smoked, and I wanted to fit in with them. I was smoking a lot. It became a horrible habit.

I finally quit for good when I was 25 years old. It was a struggle to stop smoking, and the only thing that helped me was accepting that I was hurting not only myself but also everyone around me. I had to think about all the negative effects smoking had on my appearance, my health, and even my relationships. I trained myself so well to resent smoking that now I can't be anywhere near cigarettes because smoking bothers me so much.

Smoking is a terrible habit, but good or bad, our habits help define who we are. Consistently working out and sticking to a healthful diet—with some indulgences here and there—are routines that must become habitual as we slowly but surely progress. Often this requires a paradigm shift, especially for those who are just starting out. Instead of just focusing on what we see in the mirror or on the scale, we need to form a bigger picture of ourselves. Longevity, disease prevention, and our emotional and mental health are all factors that are positively and dramatically affected by making a habit out of our healthy routines. How we look is just icing on the cake!

When Motivation Fades

Motivation is great, and working out when you're inspired is awesome. But what about when you're exhausted and hungry and the last thing you want to do is work out? That's when you rely on your habits, and that's why it's so important to create healthy habits for yourself. Many times in your fitness journey, you will be less motivated than you are right now as you read this book. That's why you need to make working out and eating well habits. Motivation alone can't dictate whether you work out today, tomorrow, or next week—not if you want to be successful. I liken working out to brushing my teeth. Did you know that most people in the United States didn't start brushing their teeth daily until the dawn of commercial television in the 1940s? Suddenly they were bombarded with commercials beaming out white teeth. Folks needed to buy toothpaste and start brushing their teeth daily if they wanted one of those gorgeous smiles. People were motivated to *start* brushing their teeth by those amazing ads, but then they kept doing it because it became a daily habit. When you brush your teeth now, are you doing it because you want beautiful teeth or because it's just what you do before you go to bed? Exactly. Exercise is the same way. It should be treated with the same consistency as your personal hygiene.

Consistency Trumps Motivation

At ZGYM, I constantly remind my members that consistency trumps motivation. Consistency means blasting through another set of burpees or squats when your mind is telling you that it wants to quit. There will often be days, even weeks, where motivation will be hard to find and fatigue a constant unwanted companion. That is when it's *crucial* that we put our heads down, grit our teeth, and blast through our workouts. Being able to work out during those periods may seem terrible and daunting, but it will make you both physically and mentally stronger. And that strength will carry over into your daily life. There is a psychological response of feeling better after a workout, and the more you can do—or the better you perform—the better you feel about yourself. The feeling or perception of doing well and doing something good for your body also can lead you to exercise more frequently or for longer or both.

So you need a spark of motivation. You need to form habits that will carry you through those stretches when your enthusiasm wanes. You can create any habit you want and eventually fall in love with it, no matter how hard it seems right now. You just have to start now and push yourself through the first month before you can expect it to feel comfortable. Most of us who exercise on a regular basis already know that once we become consistent, working out becomes second nature. No longer does it feel like a chore or a punishment but rather a part of our typical day, one that we look forward to. In fact, missing more than a day makes us feel as though something is missing in our lives. Personally, I'm at the point where it's impossible for me *not* to exercise, even if it's just a five-minute workout. I simply must, and if that's an addiction, then it's a healthy addiction.

Following a consistent routine is the most important factor when it comes to changing your body. You have to do your workouts and maintain a healthy diet on a regular basis. It's also important to remember that you can't just change your body overnight. You have to stick with your program and be honest about your efforts. Eat right daily and give 100 percent in every workout and I promise you will see and feel the difference!

Forming Positive Habits

At this point, you're probably asking, "OK, Zuzka, so how do I form habits?" Well, if you're like most people, you've been forming them your entire life. Unfortunately, many of those habits have been unhealthy. You might habitually hit the snooze button on your alarm clock three times before getting out of bed. You might habitually enter the fast-food drive-through lane at lunch instead of cooking a nutritious meal, packing it, and bringing it to work. You might habitually go to bed two hours later than you should . . . which might explain your love affair with the snooze button.

As I mentioned at the start of the chapter, I used to be a chain smoker, a habit that I eventually broke. Another bad habit of mine was pouring sugar into my favorite beverages. I trained myself and created a new habit that turned into personal preference: I now drink my tea and coffee unsweetened.

Whether you want to lose weight, add muscle, gain strength, or boost your energy, your habits will determine your success. Most of your vices are practiced behaviors, and I need you to start practicing the behaviors of working out and eating right. Habits form in the same way you exercise. You do a workout, your muscles grow, and you become stronger.

People who work out are happier than those who don't, so once developed, the habit of working out is easily reinforced. A study conducted at Stanford University over ten years reported lower depressive symptoms among exercisers in subsequent years of follow-up. In addition, those who reported more exercise had a lower incidence of concurrent depression, despite negative life events or ongoing medical problems. This justifies the need for exercise in maintaining a healthy, happy lifestyle. Physiologically, exercise stimulates the release of endorphins (serotonin, epinephrine, and dopamine), which all provide a feeling of euphoria and pain reduction, according to A. H. Goldfarb, PhD, and his colleague at the University of North Carolina at Greensboro.

Working out is now a habit for me, and so is the way I work out. I love working out at home and doing short intense circuits because it's been working for me for seven years. I just don't like going to the gym. I wouldn't change that for anything, because working out at home makes me feel comfortable. I consider that to be a positive thing that improves my life. When is the best time for you to work out? It might help you form the habit if you train at the same time every day. Others might find this too restrictive, and for those people, rigidity might keep them from working out.

Excuses, Excuses

So what keeps us mired in the bad habits and prevents us from developing good habits instead? Often it's excuses. Here is one I hear all the time: "I don't have time to work out and eat healthy." All the more reason to make this lifestyle habitual. Normally I aim for a 15-minute workout, but if I'm really busy, I'll shrink it to as little as 5 minutes. But I don't skip working out, just in the same way I would never skip taking my shower.

Another typical excuse is "I can't focus on my own fitness because I am a parent." Well, you need to accept that you are going to be so much more empowered and have such a huge advantage because parenting is so much easier if your body is strong and healthy and gets good exercise.

Try tuning out any kind of negative emotional response and treat exercise like you do your job. We often go to work and run errands with little enthusiasm and motivation, and yet we still do these things, partly out of responsibility, but also because we know they are necessary. Diet and exercise are no different. We are responsible for our well-being, and nothing plays a greater role in that than our fitness.

Without a committed approach, excuses can quickly undermine our resolve to be fit. Parvinder Punia, a British-born ZGYM member who now lives in the Czech Republic, my homeland, says:

> I think excuses are what we make ourselves, not what others project onto us. I have no family support, a full-time job that involves travel, a baby, and a boyfriend who works and trains as much as I do. My boyfriend and I just make our body a priority. At age 35 I learned swimming and started road

biking while continuing with my running. When my baby was born, I was 44 pounds overweight, tired, and suffering from backaches. Thanks to Zuzka's workouts, I lost all of it and more by the time baby was seven months! I did workouts during every nap she took; by eight weeks I had run five miles again . . . and by 11 weeks I was back on my first road ride. I was hoping I could do 15 miles, but I ended up doing 24!

How to Snap Out of Negative Thinking

Sometimes, no matter how hard we try to stay positive, negative thoughts can creep into our mind. If they become persistent enough, your entire mood can change. Here are some strategies to address negative thinking before it begins to affect various aspects of your life, including your health and fitness.

1. Get Outdoors

Something about exposure to fresh air, sunshine, and nature clears the mind and casts our problems in a new light, and that's true whether you live in the country, the suburbs, or the city. My boyfriend, Jesse, and I love taking our dogs out for walks in Los Angeles—I find it to be therapeutic and great for my emotional well-being. Being outdoors is also a perfect setting for running, yoga, and other forms of stretching, but it can be therapeutic even if all you do is walk around and breathe deeply. Sunshine offers very specific health benefits too. Many people are deficient in vitamin D, which is important for cardiovascular and bone health as well as other health properties. Sunshine is a great source of free D.

2. Take a Shower

Showers are important not just for hygiene but also as a tool for recuperation and restoration. If you think about it, a nice warm shower is the simplest form of massage. I don't know about you, but I often find that much of my stress goes away as the water runs off my skin, especially after a workout. I experience not only physical relaxation but also mental relaxation. In fact, as my brain activity gets quieter in the shower or immediately afterward, I often solve problems that I couldn't before. I can't tell you how many of my aha moments have come in the shower.

3. Listen to Music

I'm always amazed at the power of music not just to motivate me for workouts but also to take my mind off negative thoughts when I'm feeling down. Music is used to soothe human beings from infancy through palliative care settings and everywhere in between. What works for one person may not work for another. My tastes are eclectic when it comes to music. I can listen to anything. When I'm really trying to relax, I play ambient chill-out music.

4. Learn to Be Grateful

We all struggle in life sometimes, but sometimes we pay too much attention to the bad things and too little to the good. If you feel frustrated and overwhelmed because you're overweight and out of shape, remind yourself that you have the capacity to

change as long as you are healthy enough to move about and exercise. Not everyone has that privilege. Gratitude can help lessen stress and depressive symptoms. In my own life, I've found that learning to be thankful for whatever might be is hugely important!

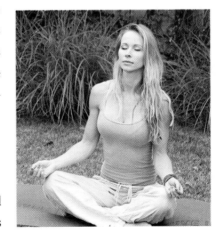

5. Stop Blaming Yourself

Are you your own most vocal critic? That kind of negative self-talk can put you in a rut that's hard to escape. Stop beating yourself up over every little thing. For example, instead of always focusing on what's wrong with your body, learn to appreciate what's great about your body.

6. Change Your Circumstances

At times when I've felt down, changing my environment has been helpful. You may need your friends to help you do this, so don't hesitate to reach out. It's almost like you need people to drag you out and take you on a vacation. If you're down, there's probably something in your life that's making you feel that way. If you stay in the same old routines, it's hard to escape the blues.

7. Work Out!

My favorite antidote to the blues is to get moving! One reason exercise is so effective at helping you snap out of negative thinking is that it makes you active and in control instead of passive and at the mercy of whatever happens to be dogging you. There are also biochemical changes that occur when we exercise that work against feeling negative and depressed.

Before Moving On to the Next Chapter

So the goal is to stay in a positive mind-set rather than a negative one, the sort of mental space that allows for good habits to be sustained and bad habits to be avoided. As part of this, I want you to experience 15 minutes of truly deep relaxation. My relaxation routine is just as short and effective as my workouts. If you can mix this into your routine two or three times a week, you'll feel amazing.

Step 1: Drink Homemade Herbal Tea

Make yourself a special, stress-relieving tea. A chamomile and ginger blend is a natural source of calm and relaxation. I suggest whole dried chamomile flowers, which can be found at farmers' markets, specialty tea shops, and even well-stocked grocery stores. I use 3 to 4 whole dried chamomile flowers and a 1½-inch piece of peeled fresh ginger cut into ¼-inch disks. I add them to 4 cups of boiling water, turn off the heat, and let the mixture steep for about 5 minutes until the water becomes infused with the blend of soothing, spicy flavors. Strain the tea, then breathe in the aroma and sip away your worries, the healthy way.

Step 2: Take a Detox Bath

While your tea is steeping, start preparing your detox bath with Epsom salts. My favorite kind is pharmaceutical-grade lavender-scented Epsom salts. I add 1 cup of salts to my bath for deep relaxation. The health benefits of these salts have been known for hundreds of years and include relaxing the nervous system, relieving inflammation, easing pain, and clearing up skin problems. This is the perfect antidote to sore muscles, which you may experience during the first week of my 30-day program.

The benefits of Epsom salts are not just skin deep, however. It's absorbed through the skin and replenishes your body's magnesium levels, which are sometimes low in people who are stressed out. Magnesium is known to create a feeling of calm by helping produce serotonin, a mood-elevating chemical that enhances the sense of deep relaxation. You can also make your own detox beauty scrub out of Epsom salts, as it has an amazing healing and soothing effect on your skin and complexion.

I sip the tea during my 20-minute bath. You have to try it!

Step 3: Nourish Your Mind

Whether it's in a nice cup of tea or a relaxing warm tub, I easily find my way to nirvana with these methods. Listening to peaceful and soothing background music

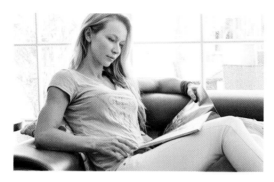

when I take a bath also increases my serenity. This can be a time to reflect on life by either giving thanks or realizing the need for change. It's important that no matter what you do, do things that make you happy. That is why I enjoy this time to myself. Most of our daily activities are for our kids, our siblings, our parents, our friends, our employer—but not for ourselves. It's crucial that you start putting yourself first on more than rare occasions, and that you start treating yourself with the love and care you give to others. You have to take care of your mind and body so that they take care of you.

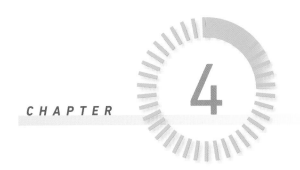

The Magic of Accountability

T his may surprise you, but I believe a lot of women and men will buy this book and keep it under wraps, as if they were holding a secret. I can see them bringing it home and not even telling their friends and family members they've just started exercising. This very common insecurity reflects the intimidation factor that often accompanies working out for the first time. Perhaps they expect to fail. Perhaps they think others will expect them to fail and will laugh at them for even trying. They may have tried before, only to end up back where they started. No one wants to subject himself or herself to that sort of ridicule. Easier just to try again in secret, in hopes of defying expectations.

At a certain point, though, I want you to become accountable to others for your health and fitness. I want you to tell friends, family, and colleagues you are committing to be fit. I want you to write about your training and diet on social media networks like Facebook, Twitter, and Instagram. You certainly don't need to tell everyone every time you enter the gym, or share every recipe you make before eating it, but you should definitely join social media conversations. This will reinforce your enthusiasm when things are going well—fueling the fire, as it were—but it may be even more important when your enthusiasm flags, and believe me, at some point your enthusiasm will flag. It happens to everyone. Picture this: It's freezing and rainy, and you're under the covers with your dog and a pile of chocolate, but your friend is waiting for you at the park for some outdoor burpees. The thought of your friend waiting all alone in the freezing rain might be the only thing that propels you out of bed on this day. In those moments, your accountability to others may be just what's needed to keep going rather than giving up.

This chapter is about establishing strong connections with others, managing the relationships you already have, and maybe even breaking some bonds if necessary. I believe all of us are fundamentally social beings. It doesn't mean we don't need our alone time—I know I do—but early humans didn't live alone unless it was a form of punishment. In the same way our brain evolved to support our bodies' movement, it evolved to enable us to share our experiences, not hold them under lock and key.

You will be less likely to achieve the goals outlined in this book if you don't forge strong relationships with others. I want to encourage you to find an "accountability" (training) partner or to form a group (a book group or a Meetup, for example) to tackle your health challenges together. You can see this when you visit my website. None of us is an island when it comes to health and fitness; we're all in this together.

Your Spheres of Influence

When you start my program, some people will encourage you, some people will be distractions, and some people may even seek to undermine you out of their own insecurities. In one way or another, people influence your journey for better or worse. Just think about our fitness "relationship." Chances are good that if you picked up this book, you have trained while viewing one of my YouTube videos at some point in the past. You and I weren't occupying the same space for the workout, but I was instructing you and offering encouragement nonetheless. We were virtual workout partners that day, perhaps for many days.

Some people can be active obstacles in your journey to fitness. The first person to discourage me was my mother, because she never wanted me to do anything active when I was growing up. She harbored health concerns that I now realize were greatly exaggerated, and it took me years to get over her disapproval and to teach myself to work out. I had nobody in my corner and started all by myself, and it was *hard*. I highly recommend finding yourself a support system.

So who should you train with? The ideal training partner should have goals that resemble, if not match, your own. If you're trying to lose 40 pounds and partner up with somebody who wants to turn into She-Hulk, the workout relationship probably won't end happily. You and your partner also should have similar preferences regarding workout times. If you can't stand exercising before work in the morning, and that's the only time your partner can train, the two of you are likely headed for a training-partner divorce at some point fairly soon.

When the pairing works well, though, training partners are awesome. On those days when you don't feel like working out, you'll be more likely to train anyway because someone is counting on you, and you won't want to let him or her down. This is one of the reasons many people hire a personal trainer. More than the instruction they will receive, clients no longer have a choice whether to show up; otherwise, they have to cancel and most likely pay for a session they didn't attend, which is a waste of money.

The quality of your workout often skyrockets with a good training partner because the two of you can push each other to train harder. One can motivate the other to finish one last rep, smashing through preconceived limitations in the process. Training partners or training groups can make working out more fun than solo sessions would allow. You can compare times, turning your workouts into challenges, which I absolutely love.

You can learn from your training partner, too, by trading ideas back and forth regarding diet, workouts, supplements, and other facets of fitness. During the workout, you and your partner can also keep an eye on each other's form, correcting it as needed. You don't need to be a certified personal trainer to tell someone, "Hey, your hips are sagging when you do planks!" or "Your knees are getting out in front of your feet when you do squats!"

The best training partners are as invested in your success as they are in their own, and they should feel the same support from you. They show up a few minutes early and are ready to go when the workout starts. They don't vent about their crappy day or the fight they just had with their significant other; instead, they come armed with positive vibes and contagious energy. They celebrate when you crush a new goal. Nobody wants to be around someone selfish, and that applies to workout settings. If your partner whines and complains, and doesn't have the courtesy to let you know in advance when she can't train that day—leaving you waiting 10 or 15 minutes before starting on your own—she is more hindrance than help. Cut her loose before her bad habits rub off on you.

Finding Support for Fitness

Whether you train with a partner, a group, or alone, your interactions with people will affect you once you've nailed your workout and changed out of your sweats. If you have a significant other, his or her reaction to what you're doing could influence not only your success but also the relationship itself. Couples who shape up together— or at least support each other in this endeavor—may find that their relationship grows even stronger along with their bodies. Yet another scenario can unfold. Namely, one partner starts shaping up and the other partner greets those efforts with apathy or even disdain and ridicule.

It's sad to think that would ever happen, but I'm telling you, it occurs more often than you might believe. Sometimes people who don't work out feel bad about being out of shape, and seeing their partners succeed when they haven't casts their own insecurities and shortcomings in a harsh light. Relationships can grow even more tense when the ones who *are* shaping up start getting, shall we say, noticed more than before. Other people start checking them out, and if it happens when their partner is nearby, imagine what happens when they are alone. This often becomes a crossroads in the relationship. If you're the one who isn't shaping up, will you step up your game or at least encourage rather than discour-

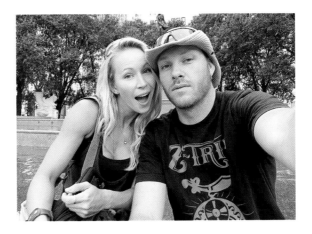

age your partner? If not, are you prepared to lose him or her? The risk is there. The one thing I've learned for sure through my experiences is that a major lifestyle change reveals your true friends. They will be the ones *supporting* you, not the ones trying to hold you back or drag you down.

I'm not saying you need to be one of those couples joined at the hip in the gym, either. In fact, you may not even enjoy the same fitness activities, which is fine. What matters is that you're both passionate about fitness and your health and that you both want to bring new energy and interesting experiences back to the relationship. That's how it worked out for one of my followers, Sophia.

When my husband and I were first married, I was a runner. I tried to get my husband to run with me, but he hated every second of it, which would also make me miserable running with him. Over time, we discovered that he loves hiking, biking, and manual labor—namely farming—and I love high-intensity interval training, yoga, and lifting weights. Sometimes we work out together but usually separately. We encourage each other and give each other the time and equipment we need to stay healthy. The biggest thing for me was listening to him and helping him find what he loved instead of getting him to do what I love.

Five Ways to Motivate Your Significant Other Without Being a Jerk

Whether it's your husband or your wife, your boyfriend or your girlfriend, it can be hard, even annoying, to watch your partner continually veg out in front of the television with a bag of potato chips while you work your butt off to shape up. Every relationship requires compromise, and you each need to respect each other's habits and space. Beyond that, here are some tips for navigating this potential minefield.

1. Build Her Up, Don't Break Her Down

Any attempts at motivating your partner need to come with love and out of a genuine concern for her health. Guilt and put-downs are the two worst things you can offer a partner who doesn't have much motivation to exercise or commit to a healthier lifestyle; they create only animosity and resentment. Instead, try to find positive methods to gently nudge your significant other toward fitness and health.

2. Don't Give Ultimatums

As with guilt and put-downs, ultimatums do not motivate people to work out unless something immediately threatens their health. Don't tell your partner that affection of any kind will be withheld unless she gets off her lazy butt or something to that effect. At best, ultimatums may provide a short-term solution, but fitness and wellbeing are all about the long haul. A gentle, positive nudging every so often will go a lot further than nagging.

3. Work Out Together

Do simple activities together that involve both of you working out. Try bike rides or hikes. Long walks can be a good way to start out as well. Maybe your significant other may not be at your level of fitness yet, but gently nurturing her toward fitness and making it fun can make all the difference in convincing her to work out consistently.

4. Set Goals Together

Time your walks, runs, or hikes. Over the course of a few weeks of consistently working out together, see if you can beat your previous times or go a little farther than before. Goal setting provides a great deal of motivation, especially when the goal, however small it may be, is achieved. Positive reinforcement really works and goal setting together can provide positive growth in any relationship.

5. Focus on Health, Not Appearance

This is really important, especially if your partner is out of shape or overweight. Make sure her health, not how she looks, is the priority. Focusing on looks can often make a person self-conscious and, worse, incredibly insecure. It also makes her feel as though your affection and attraction for her are based only on her physical appearance, not on who she is as a complete person. This, of course, is counterproductive for a healthy, lasting relationship.

The workplace is another social setting that may play a huge role in your fitness success or failure. As with your spouse, some coworkers may offer support, and some may heap on the hate, especially if they're jealous of your progress. Your work environment can be especially hard on your diet. If the break room always has a box of doughnuts on the countertop, you may find yourself mindlessly indulging with your morning coffee. When you join a group of colleagues for lunch, they're probably not going to look for the cleanest meals in town, opting for speed and convenience instead. After work, happy hour is another diet trap.

If you're lucky, your workplace can become part of your support system. Some companies have cafeterias that prepare nutritious, inexpensive food. Corporate gyms, or at least reimbursement for gym memberships, are now commonplace all over the country. Some companies reimburse employees for riding their bike to work. Cycling is both a great cardiovascular workout and an environmentally friendly mode of commuting.

Over the years, I've worked with only one other person, a videographer who produces my workout videos, so I don't have much experience working in large companies of the sort I just described. However, my coauthor, Jeff O'Connell, is the editor in chief of Bodybuilding.com, which is a model for companies that support health and fitness among their employees. When you walk through the front door in Boise, Idaho, the first thing you see is a large, well-equipped gym buzzing with activity. Before work, during lunch, or after work, people are arrayed on the cardio machines, and unused free weights are in short supply. The company also does employee transformation challenges and has on-staff trainers to help employees reach their fitness goals. Beyond what the company does, though, it's the amazing support among employees that makes these efforts so successful. For a person who is getting in shape, bringing a healthy meal to meetings and skipping doughnuts in the break room isn't the outlier at Bodybuilding.com; it's the norm. On occasion you might see a person or two outside in the designated smoking area, but they look really lonely.

My point is that your environment will play a role in all of this, even if you're training at home and keeping your fitness goals quiet. So do your best to make your environment one that's conducive to wellness. Get a training buddy, toss out your secret cookie stash, and join an online community where people will be psyched about your accomplishments. There's no need to be at the mercy of your surroundings!

Find Your Fitness Community

One thing that can make fitness fun is the sense of being part of a community, one that goes beyond a workout partner or friends and family or even your workplace. In my opinion, that's why CrossFit has been so successful: People go to their "box" for a kick-butt workout, to be sure, but they're also drawn to a community of like-minded people. What's more, they love competing with their friends and fellow CrossFitters. It's their fitness activity and their sport rolled into one.

If you're not into CrossFit, consider taking up a sport like golf, basketball, or tennis. I don't know anyone who would say, "Oh my God, I have to go play tennis today.

Geez, I hate it so much." I've never heard a football player talking about his hatred of playing his sport. People are always excited when there are competitive aspects to their exercise.

Regardless of which sport or activity you pursue, building more muscle and stamina through fitness will make it both easier and more fun. And as we become more productive and happier while exercising, our enthusiasm and willingness to try new and challenging things also increase. When you're in great shape you can not only start doing a different workout in the gym or at home but also enjoy more outdoor activities like hiking, kayaking, tennis, or even rock climbing. Nothing will prevent you from joining a random sports game and you will be able to accept any challenges from now on.

So find a sport or any physical activity that you've always wanted to try. Or maybe you used to do something when you were younger and stopped for lack of time, family issues, or some other reason. Now it's the time to reinvent yourself, to be more adventurous, to try something new. I'm sure you can think of some sport that you very well might excel at—something that will make you feel proud and passionate. The possibilities are endless! The point is not to reach the professional level but to have fun, stay active, and be social.

Just as important as getting into better shape, you can meet new friends and become part of something bigger than yourself. One more thing: Do *not* wait until you get into shape to start with a sport. That's the number one excuse for most people who are avoiding a new or once-practiced activity. Don't be afraid of judgment. Don't be afraid that others will laugh at you because you're a little clumsy or overweight. *Right this minute, stop caring what anyone thinks!* Being a good person with a positive mind-set is way more important than your looks or sport skills. Everyone who thinks differently can kiss your rear end. You're a Warrior!

One of my followers, Kathleen, found her calling in pounding the pavement. "I'm committing to meeting up with a local running group every Tuesday night," she wrote. "We do a short three-mile run and then socialize afterward at a local restaurant and bar. I always have fun and I've met great people."

Stay Fit with Fido

This may surprise you, but your pets can play an important role in your health, fitness, and happiness. Any of you who visit my website know animals are very important to me and my boyfriend, Jesse. Along with working on my website, Jesse is an accomplished animal trainer. We have four dogs: two mastiffs, one Doberman pinscher, and a rat terrier. So we have all different shapes and sizes. They all have different personalities too. We put them in the car and take them to the wash along the Los Angeles River, where they can run around with other dogs and move about freely. I love their companionship. They're like family to me.

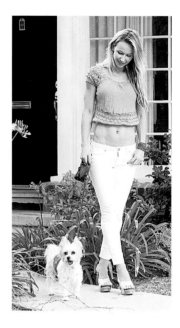

Your pets may drive you crazy sometimes, but they do something else: They keep you active. When you take them out for a walk or jog, they're not the only ones getting in a workout. A study out of Michigan State University reported that, on average, pet owners were 34 percent more physically active than their non-pet-owning counterparts and were more likely to get in the American College of Sports Medicine (ACSM) and American Heart Association (AHA)–recommended 150-plus minutes of moderate-intensity exercise per week. Granted, the canines may need little breaks to do their business and perhaps sniff around, but they are often the ones encouraging their owners to take them out for a walk.

> *Until one has loved an animal, a part of one's soul remains unawakened.*
>
> —ANATOLE FRANCE

Don't forget, your pet needs the exercise too. It's shocking, but more than half of all pets in the United States are overweight or obese. Gives new meaning to the notion of dogs looking like their masters—and obesity creates the same sort of health problems in pets that it does in humans. There are even fitness trackers for pets now!

Woman's (and Man's) Best Friend

Pets are great for boosting your mood and releasing stress. In the previous chapter, I told you exercise is linked to fewer symptoms of depression, and now you know owning a dog can increase your amount of physical activity. So owning a dog is good for your physical and mental health.

Several studies have reported the additive effect of dog ownership on physical and psychological well-being. One study in particular was conducted out of the University of Warwick in Coventry, UK, where researchers reported the dog-led facilitation of social interaction improved overall well-being. In addition, research in the mid-1990s reported that dogs' sense of loyalty and companionship reduced symptoms of depression and improved mood in adult college students. I'm a firm believer that the better your mood and the less stress you have, the more likely you are to stick with your workouts and diet.

Finally, pets are an excellent way to meet people. Any guy knows that if he's walking a cute dog, women will stop and fawn over his pet, creating a perfect opening for interaction. The same goes if a woman is walking the dog. Pets are one of the best icebreakers ever, so get your pet and get outside! Walking your pet can coexist on the same days as all the workouts in the book, and it really makes a perfect active rest activity.

Posting as Luci, one of my followers talked about the role her pet played in her fitness. "I'm gonna start walking again with my dog! He's been at a friend's house because my place was too small, but it's time to get my walking partner! He loves to be first, so walks turn into runs!"

Social Media

Today it's almost impossible to separate fitness from social media. Every time you're on Facebook, Instagram, Pinterest, or Twitter, you're likely to see selfies of your friends' physiques, pictures of their healthy recipes, and "fitspirational" memes saying "Strong is the next sexy" or "Sweat is just fat crying." I'm a huge user of social media myself. I got my start posting videos on YouTube, and today I post on Facebook, Twitter, Instagram, and elsewhere as often as I can.

Yes, many people portray an idealized version of themselves and their life on social media. I don't know anyone who posts their failures or their worst photographs, at least not voluntarily. When it's you and your life, you know about failures all too well. We all do. I used to be inspired by photos of bodies of the sort you see on social media all day, but that faded as my source of inspiration. As I mentioned earlier, now I'm more inspired by athletes reaching their goals. More superficial forms of motivation didn't last for me.

I also find social media to be a great source of useful information. When people share recipes—that's the best. That's awesome. I also look for new exercises on social media. I may see something intriguing and tweak it with my own Z spin.

At the end of the day, it's important to be happy for the success of others, and not to see it as proof of your shortcomings. If I see someone else being successful, it doesn't fill my heart with envy; it fills my heart with hope and happiness. If you can be successful, then I can be successful too. If you are happy, I can be happy too, and I like to watch how you did it, because it inspires me. I truly *love* to see people succeed! It pushes me to keep reaching for my own goals and dreams, and to never, ever give up.

CHAPTER   5

Fuel for Your Workouts, Medication for Your Moods

There it is. That last piece of your husband's birthday cake. You already indulged the night before, but this one last piece has been taunting you all day at work. In fact, it even tried seducing you last night while you were trying to sleep. This cake is fifty shades of delicious. You come home after a long workday to your sugar, and your husband, and you don't know which one you'd rather take a bite out of first. Actually, you do. Who are we kidding? That's chocolate frosting. This is impossible to resist.

Almost. You can, and you will, fight the temptation because you are stronger than a few bites of chocolate cake. The satisfaction of not picking up that fork will be worth it when you can finally pick up a size smaller pair of jeans and finally wear a new bikini to the beach!

Without a doubt, the battle between self-control and instant gratification can feel as epic as David versus Goliath. It can be daunting, to say the least, especially when it comes to fitness and well-being. Do not—I repeat—*do not* consider a sudden, compulsive need for instant gratification in the form of doughnuts, cheeseburgers, cake, or pizza to be a character flaw, a lack of willpower, or a sign that something is genuinely

47

lacking inside of you. Instead, consider it a form of mismanaging stress, priorities, and the goals you've set for yourself. That's it. In other words, don't make it a personal issue or the fault of God or the cosmos. That kind of thinking often leads to a downward spiral that forges a negative self-image. In turn, a negative self-image leads to—you guessed it—a craving for instant gratification.

Certain foods can trigger moods and dictate our overall energy. They can be used as medicine for our body and mind. If abused, they can also lead to addiction and health problems. Perhaps the greatest trigger that leads us to leap impulsively over restaurant counters and devour a tray of doughnuts is chronic stress. When stress is a constant in our lives, our minds and bodies begin to short-circuit. This can have a huge impact on your hormones, and hormones control *everything*! If you've ever been around a pregnant woman, you know this already. As with so many health-related issues, stress is multifactorial, but to put it simply: When stress locks in, the brain sends a signal to release a cascade of effects on glands that produce hormones. Eventually, cortisol is released by the adrenal glands. Cortisol is considered a stress hormone. It is usually released in our bodies during moments of anxiety and stress, including depression.

This is one example among many other effects. A study conducted at Harvard University reported that whereas short-term stress can actually suppress appetite, chronic stress has the opposite effect, guiding people to "comfort" foods that tend to be high in calories and laden with unhealthy fats. The more stress present, the more an individual tends to indulge, according to the authors of the Harvard study.

Emotional eating is a phrase heard often. It refers to someone binging on junk food high in unhealthy fats and processed sugar for days or even weeks due to stress or anxiety. The truth is that emotional eating, or stress eating, plays a significant role in the obesity epidemic and can also be an indication of deeper, more dangerous disorders. Research from the early 1990s first started to evaluate the close ties between overeating and weight gain and how stress seemed to be the overlying problem. In 2007, a study conducted at Deakin University in Australia concluded that under the condition of chronic stress, individuals are enticed to consume high-energy (caloric-dense) food and the additional calories consumed are not available to be used as energy but rather are stored as excess fat.

Recent research by the American Psychological Association demonstrated a very strong link between stress and weight gain. What's more, a recent Harvard study indicated that women were more likely to turn to food when stressed, whereas men were more likely to use smoking and alcohol as a coping mechanism. An extensive study of 37,161 Finnish women and 8,649 men was in agreement with the Harvard study.

Aside from stress and anxiety, another factor that may contribute to emotional eating is our unhealthy desire to be perfect. A study out of the University of North Carolina demonstrated that women who felt a greater need to be perfect were also more likely to binge on junk food. People who obsess over trying to create a "perfect" body image predispose themselves to body dysmorphia. No matter what they do, their body will never be ideal in their eyes. This can prompt many other problems, one of which is the occasional treat—but it typically doesn't stop with one bite. There is an overindulgence and then, almost always, a punishment for doing so, such as overexercising or even purging, according to a study by the American Psychiatric Association.

Reaching for comfort foods every once in a while is perfectly OK, but when we do it habitually to compensate for negative feelings or to counter the effects of stress or anxiety, it becomes a problem. When stress is coupled with an unhealthy fixation on body image, it can even lead to eating disorders such as bulimia.

The Stanford Marshmallow Experiment, one of the first studies done on self-control and instant gratification, is enlightening. Performed during the 1970s by psychologist Walter Mischel, the study aimed to show the value of self-control and delayed gratification in children. Kids were offered either an immediate reward in the form of a marshmallow or a greater, more valuable reward if they chose to wait for the treat. The study demonstrated that the kids who chose to wait tended to achieve greater success later in life in the form of higher test scores and overall health.

Studies like the Marshmallow Experiment tell us that self-control and patience—even if it involves a bit of a battle within ourselves—are worth it. Why? Because you are worth it.

Don't lose weight simply to look better. It's *healthy* for your body to be in shape, and you'll feel better too! I'm now convinced that many people struggle to stay motivated because their goals are limited to staying slim and sexy—external motivation. That's not enough! We all want to feel great, which gives us the confidence we need to succeed. The food that I choose to eat is delicious, energy boosting, satisfying, and fun to share.

Before we get into the specifics of nutrition, I want to stress something: You have to eat! Some newbies in ZGYM have told me, "I'm not losing weight, but I barely eat . . ." Well, that's the problem! View food as *fuel* for your body; it's totally necessary but needs to be the right kind of stuff, and depriving your body of food is as idiotic as trying to drive on an empty tank of gas. This program isn't about starvation or deprivation. This about giving your body what it needs to work hard and look amazing.

How to Lose Weight

As you can see, the body, mind, and food are all connected. I just mentioned some of the things that cause us to eat too much or the wrong kinds of foods. So what is the right amount and what are the healthy foods, the ones that keep your body weight where it should be while keeping you energized all day? You want answers, I know.

Nutrition is an intimate part of so many aspects of our life. Any nutritionist could write up a diet full of meal plans that will work if followed to a T. But your diet doesn't exist in a vacuum; adherence depends on how you feel physically and emotionally at any moment. If you're sick and your appetite has changed, that meal plan suddenly doesn't work. If all you can stomach is saltines, you won't want your chicken and broccoli, no matter how nutritious they are. If you and your boyfriend or husband just had a fight, and you're upset, chances are you will not follow that meal plan. If you don't have access to the exact food mentioned in the diet, a substitute must be found, and it might not be as healthy a choice. If dinner calls for foods X, Y, and Z, but your friends want to go out, let's face it, the evening's meal plan is out the window. I easily could rattle off ten more scenarios that could upend your well-intentioned meal plan.

Those examples aren't dietary disasters. This is *life* unfolding. I don't want you to skip an evening out with your friends because your diet is rigid. What fun is that? Instead, I want you to learn certain habits and patterns, but in a way that allows deviation as needed before returning to your plan. The habits I'm talking about are ones like eating consistently, at three- or

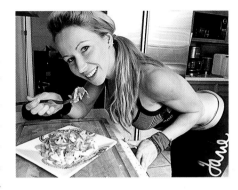

four-hour intervals, rather than feasting and then skipping meals for the rest of the day. Eating at regular intervals keeps your blood sugar steady and your energy in the on position. It also prevents binge eating.

Other important habits include learning or knowing how to cook, keeping the fridge stocked with healthy foods, working out, and drinking enough water. If you're doing those things, then the occasional cheat, like eating a piece of chocolate cake, won't kill you. You'll indulge and continue with your plan because the habits underlying it remain firmly in place. You didn't fall out of shape overnight, so you won't regain total health and fitness overnight either. Start now, though, no matter what's happening in your life. If you wait for perfect conditions, they won't ever come.

You're not dieting; you're changing your lifestyle. My lifestyle has never been better than it is now because for the first time in my life, I care about eating healthfully more than I care about being slim. My meals consist mostly of protein, veggies, and lots of healthy fats like olive oil, coconut oil, and avocados. Ironically, I am actually getting better results in terms of my body composition now that I've stopped focusing on it.

However, if you are overweight, part of becoming healthy is losing that excess weight. No doubt the desire for weight loss prompted some of you to pick up this book. Weight loss is often presented as a dizzying and complex endeavor requiring nothing short of witchcraft to accomplish. Thousands upon thousands of fad diets and trendy exercise regimens crowd the fitness landscape, and new ones pop up every month.

Weight loss is a very simple formula. Not simple to accomplish—the current obesity pandemic testifies to that fact—but weight loss boils down to mathematics. OK, are you ready? I'm about to turn you into a weight loss Jedi. The secret formula is: You must consistently consume fewer calories than your body requires and/or burn the necessary calories through exercise to create a caloric deficit. Then, and only then, will you lose weight. On page 85 you'll find a chart for specific calorie counts based on body weight.

Those calories we're talking about are simply units of energy our body uses to live and function. If the body doesn't receive the necessary amount of energy from food and drink at any given time, it will tap into other sources—namely, fat stores or muscle—for its energy needs. The goal is to burn off unwanted fat and keep hard-earned, shapely muscle. Which gets burned depends on how significant the caloric deficit is and how long it lasts. Regardless, weight loss results from a sustained calorie deficit.

The reality show *Survivor* offers a highly visual example of how a calorie deficit leads to weight loss. All of the show's contestants are required to live in some remote location and survive off the land. This food scarcity creates a sudden calorie deficit in the contestants, and they shed a considerable amount of weight over the course of the show. During the second season, Elisabeth Hasselbeck lost so much weight that her hair started to fall out. This example may be extreme, but it does get rid of a lot of the smoke and mirrors attached to weight loss.

The weight loss formula sounds simple, yet it feels anything *but* simple. Many people struggle with weight loss because it requires a great deal of discipline and work. Also, our frustrations and emotions can keep us from progressing as fast as we would like to. Even worse, sometimes our judgments of ourselves sabotage our hard work at the gym or in the kitchen.

What's more, while the formula for weight loss is simple math, there's a big difference between weight loss and healthy weight loss. Where your calories come from *matters*. Restricting yourself to 1,200 calories a day but eating them in the form of pizza and fries won't do you any favors. Healthy weight loss can be achieved by eating healthful foods in the right amounts, combined with regular exercise.

Measuring Your Macronutrients

Whether you're eating healthfully or poorly, the calories you consume will come in three forms: protein, carbohydrate, and fat. These are called macronutrients. It's important to think about the ratio in which you consume these macronutrients, whether it's 40:40:20, 36:43:21, or what have you. Let me explain a little bit about each one.

Protein

Protein is what your body uses to build stuff, whether it's your flawless skin, your silky hair, your internal organs, the muscles you flex, even your blood, in the form of hemoglobin. Protein also produces enzymes, hormones, and neurotransmitters, which allow messages to zip about your body at warp speed: *Ouch, that's hot! Move your finger away from the flame NOW!* Dietary protein can also help control body fat and free fatty acids from fat tissue such as saddlebags, chicken wings, and muffin tops. Needless to say, without enough protein, your body won't function well at all.

The first thing that might hop into your brain when I mention protein is a juicy steak, a tender chicken breast, or fresh fish. Those are great sources of protein for sure, but protein comes from numerous other foods sources, some of which might surprise you. Good sources of protein include egg whites, milk, soy protein, spirulina, whey protein, quinoa, hemp seeds, poultry, fish, and meat. You can also get complete protein in an animal-friendly way by combining grains and nuts, grains and legumes.

The rule for adequate protein intake for those of you who are doing the workouts every day is 0.64 to 0.9 gram of protein per pound of body weight per day. You don't need any more protein than that; you'll get too sexy. So if you weigh 140 pounds, you would need to consume between 89.6 and 126.0 grams of protein throughout the day. Your body needs protein at regular intervals too. Eating three to five times a day would do the trick. *When* you eat will determine where your body gets its fuel too. Specifically, eating protein before and after you ace your workouts is especially important to avoid *catabolism*, a state in which your body breaks down the muscles that you've been working so hard for, instead of using ingested calories or fat stores.

One of the many things I love about protein is that energy is necessary to digest, absorb, transport, and store it. So it not only fills you up and keeps you strong but also burns extra calories while doing so. This *thermic effect* makes protein the best macronutrient for burning body fat and losing body weight.

Fat

Many people hear the word *fat* and want to run for the hills. For years consumers were instilled with a fat phobia that could be handled only by purchasing fat-free or low-fat products in supermarkets. Back then, "fat shaming" targeted the macronutrient, not the overweight. Unfortunately, many people took that to mean that if a food package included the words *fat-free* or *low-fat*, they could eat as much of it as they wanted to and still look trim. Not! This helps explain why obesity rates in the United States soared during the low-fat craze, which is only now winding down. Much of the rest of the world followed suit, leading to, among other things, a type 2 diabetes pandemic that now affects 387 million people worldwide, according to the International Diabetes Federation.

It's important to differentiate here between body fat and dietary fat. The latter doesn't necessarily lead to the former. In fact, your body wouldn't work very well without dietary fat. Actually, it wouldn't work, period. The human body can't absorb the vitamins A, D, E, and K in the absence of fat; those vitamins won't dissolve without it. Your brain couldn't tell your hands to hold this book right now if fat weren't coating both your brain's surface and the neurons transmitting messages throughout your body. What's more, fat is essential for balancing the levels of hormones such as testosterone and estrogen in the body.

Some reasonable amount of body fat is essential, too, unless you want to walk around looking like a cadaver. The membranes of the cells that make up my, your, and everyone else's body are composed of fat, which also protects our vital organs like bubble wrap and insulates us from cold weather. It's unhealthy for most people to fall below certain body fat thresholds: 5 percent for men and 12 percent for women. Many women who fall below that number lose their monthly period. If you talk to body-builders or fitness athletes nearing physique-contest day—the time when they pose for photo shoots showing off their six-pack abs—it's like talking to zombies. Sure, they're lean, but many of them can barely string a sentence together!

Fat does pack in 9 calories per gram, making it a more concentrated source of energy than both protein and carbohydrate. "Aha," you might think. "So dietary fat is what makes folks fat." Not so fast. Back in the 1940s, a cardiologist noticed that people were getting fatter and having more heart attacks and blamed high fat intake and high cholesterol. So what did the dietary establishment do? Create low- to no-fat diets. By the 1960s this was *the* diet that cardiac patients had to follow. Commercially available foods replaced the fat with fillers and artificial sweeteners (carbohydrates). But people who ate this way didn't get any thinner, and heart attacks didn't decline. Now we know that the most successful weight loss stories come from individuals who moderate their carbohydrate consumption.

There are many kinds of fat, and they all have different effects on your health. Fats can be considered polyunsaturated, monounsaturated, or saturated. Are you going to remember which is which after you put down this book? Probably not. But what I do want you to remember is that fats take on different forms at room temperature, depending on how they are processed—which in turn influences how they affect your body and waistline. Liquid fats are usually better than solid fats. Once liquid fats are processed to include more and more hydrogen molecules, they gradually take on more solid forms, from sprayable to squeezable. The result is hydrogenated or partially hydrogenated vegetable oils, in which the liquid oil is now soft margarine or stick margarine. Saturated fats are processed to include even more hydrogen molecules. This makes them easier to use. In general, it's better to stick to the more liquid form of any fat because your body will then not have to break all the extra bonds that were created in the hydrogenation process, according to Ashley Herda at the University of Kansas (Edwards).

You've probably heard for years or decades that saturated fat is to be avoided, but research does not back that up. Several studies have found no link between the consumption of saturated fats and a higher incidence of heart disease. Monounsaturated fats such as those found in olive oil, avocados, and many nuts and seeds are good for you, as are the polyunsaturated fats found in flaxseed, walnuts, and fatty fish (such as salmon, trout, mackerel, and herring). As much as these mono- and polyunsaturated fats are good for you because they help lower your bad cholesterol, the current Recommended Dietary Allowance (RDA) is to limit total fat intake to less than 35 percent of your daily consumption of calories.

Carbohydrate

Carbohydrate is the macronutrient most of us associate with energy. We "carb up" for an endurance event or game; we don't "protein up" or "fat up." In reality, carbs play a crucial role in the immune system, reproduction, blood clotting, and growth and development. Individuals should consume sufficient amounts of carbohydrate to ward off unnecessary increases in stress hormones that can affect maintenance of normal body functions. Any onset of stress, whether from exercise or insufficient nutrient intake, exacerbates the stress hormone response, throwing all systems out of balance and diminishing performance, among other things.

Healthy sources of what I call *workout-earned carbohydrate* (I'll explain this in a bit) include whole grains, potatoes, sweet potatoes, pasta, rice, quinoa, legumes, oats, wheat, bread, chocolate and other sweets, and fruits high in sugar (such as bananas, mangoes, and pineapple). What's off-limits? You should avoid candy, cake, doughnuts, muffins, white bread, chips, fast food, pastries, and ice cream.

By most standards, my diet would be considered low carb. Most days I consume fewer than 50 grams of carbohydrate. I prefer that you consume much of your carbohydrate post-workout. During a 15-minute Z blast, your body is burning something called glycogen, the stored form of glucose. So after your workout is the time to replenish your supply so you're fueled up and ready to go for your next workout. You'll also feel pretty gassed after one of my workouts, and that influx of carbs will perk you back up.

Free Meals versus Workout-Earned Meals

Of course, except for snacking, we typically don't eat individual foods. We eat meals. When I think about nutrition, I divide my meals into two types: free meals (FMs) and workout-earned meals (WEMs). This comes from the philosophy of Precision Nutrition, for which I am certified. I have been following the control-carb diet for well over six years myself. It keeps me lean, full of energy, and strong for my workouts and day-to-day activities. I believe it will help you as well.

Free Meals

Free meals are those I don't need to pay for with a workout. These types of meals are low in carbs, mostly based around veggies, protein, and healthy fats. You can pick any of my FM recipes and enjoy them at any time of the day.

Workout-Earned Meals

According to an old saying, "Weight loss is 80 percent diet, 20 percent exercise." Another old saying goes, "What you eat in private, you wear in public." Who cares if you just worked out for two hours if you ate a burger with a large order of French fries and a milk shake afterward? The body of your dreams will remain just that: a dream.

Working out does give you more latitude with your foods selection—just not *that* much latitude. Remember, weight loss is a math equation with calories consumed on one side and calories burned on the other. Blasting through one of my 15-minute workouts burns a significant number of calories, so you can add back at least some of those calories after the workout and still be ahead on your weight loss scorecard. But there's more to it. Exercise makes your body more sensitive to the effects of insulin, the hormone responsible for ushering glucose out of your bloodstream and into cells. When too much sugar stays in your bloodstream for too long, it starts causing or at least contributing to the plaque formation indicative of cardiovascular disease. This insidious process dramatically increases your risk of having a heart attack or a stroke, which is basically a brain attack.

So whereas FMs can be consumed whether you work out or not, WEMs can be consumed only during a two-hour window after a workout. The main difference between free and workout-earned meals concerns the amount and type of carbohydrates they contain. So, compared to free meals, WEMs tend to be higher in carbs, and those carbs can have a higher glycemic index (GI), meaning they break down into blood glucose faster than lower-GI carbs. Remember, though, this is the time when your insulin sensitivity is highest, and your body is at its most effective in terms of regulating your blood sugar. When you work out will determine when you consume your workout-earned meals. If I don't do my workout, I don't have these types of meals. Neither should you.

Why Detox Diets Are a Bad Idea

Some people resort to crash diets that are often deceptively called "detox" or "cleanse" diets. I know many women, and even some men, who insist they are detoxing for health purposes when, in reality, they are looking for a quick way to lose 5 to 10 pounds.

Detox diets usually last a week to a month and involve a minimal amount of eating. Women are basically told to starve themselves, except for drinking an herbal concoction to rid their bodies of harmful toxins. The most obvious example is the Master Cleanse—a famous detox diet that involves drinking a combination of lemon juice, cayenne pepper, maple syrup, and salt, followed by a laxative tea in the evening.

Detox sounds healthy; so does *cleanse*. And this is true if you're cutting back on sugar and alcohol. However, these types of diets are counterproductive to our overall health and well-being and can even be harmful. Unfortunately, as with all crash diets, the weight comes right back once you return to normal eating habits. Typical side effects of a detox diet are dizziness, fatigue, and nausea.

So if the weight loss isn't healthy or sustainable, what about the detox element? At a minimum, little scientific evidence supports these claims. Your body is incredibly efficient at getting rid of toxins on its own. The main problem is that we constantly consume unhealthy foods like added sugar. So don't go to extremes; just eat healthier.

The Surprising Truth About the Sweet Stuff

One thing I have totally cut out of my diet, workout or not, is added sugar. We all have a love–hate relationship with the sweet stuff. I'm sure you've heard sayings like "All things in moderation," "A little bit won't hurt," and "It's fuel for the brain." But the question is, should added sugar ever be consumed, and how bad is it, actually, for your health?

Pretty bad, as it turns out. Sugar contains no nutrients, no protein, and no healthy fats or enzymes—just empty, quickly digested calories. Doctors give patients 70 grams in liquid form as a metabolic stress test if they suspect impaired glucose tolerance that may or may not rise to the level of type 2 diabetes. They want to judge the patient's glucose control in the face of a blast of pure sugar. These 70 grams happen to be the same amount found in two 12-ounce cans of cola. The ready access to sugary foods has played a big role in the pandemic of obesity and other lifestyle-related diseases plaguing every country on Earth now.

When I warn you about the health risks associated with too much added sugar, I should highlight the word *added*. I'm *not* asking you to avoid fruit and vegetables, which also contain sugar. The sugars found naturally in fruit and vegetables are balanced by the fiber, vitamins, enzymes, and other properties that slow digestion and help the body deal with it more easily. Fruits, alongside vegetables, are an essential and tasty part of your diet. The benefits of eating whole fruit outweigh the small increase in carbs they may contribute to your diet. *Whole* is a key word here. Fruit juice removes many of those benefits I mentioned, including fiber. An orange and a glass of orange juice are not the same thing.

Added sugar leaves you with nothing but fleeting energy, a paunch, and maybe some zits. Those are just the effects you can immediately feel. Regular consumption of too much added sugar also stresses the liver; increases levels of unhealthy cholesterol; and can help lead to weight gain, anxieties, cravings, and disturbed sleep. A study by the U.S. Centers for Disease Control and Prevention (CDC) looked at the relationship between added sugar consumption and heart disease, and what the researchers found is pretty frightening. The average American diet contains enough added sugar to increase the risk of heart-related death by 18 percent. What's

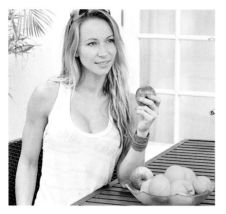

worse, consuming more than 21 percent of your calories (that's 420 calories of a 2,000-calorie-a-day diet) from added sugar more than doubles your risk of death from heart disease. Research has shown that overdoing it on the sweet stuff also can lead to obesity, type 2 diabetes, a gradual diminution of cognitive function (perhaps involving Alzheimer's), and even certain cancers.

Some of you may find that you are actually addicted to sugar, which is now a very real problem for many people. If so, I have the perfect antidote: *exercise*! Sugar raises serotonin and dopamine levels, which can factor into your cravings. Exercise can do the same thing. Try exercising when you have sugar cravings—get that rush and build your habits around that. Get addicted to the high you can get from exercise.

If the cravings persist, eat a piece of fruit. Yes, if you eat enough of it, fruit can affect your blood sugar; it does contain sugar, after all. But generally fruit will cause less of a blood sugar spike compared to nutrient-void table sugar or a cookie. A cookie may contain the same type of sugar (fructose) as a bowl of strawberries, but they are worlds apart in terms of their nutritional value and, more important, in how your body digests and processes the fructose. For one thing, strawberries are high in vitamin C, potassium, and antioxidants, and they contain fiber. This allows the liver to process the fructose at a much slower, healthier rate than the way it processes the sugars from sweets and sodas. In contrast, an average cookie contains a ridiculously high amount of artificially processed sugar and has no real nutritional value.

Also, the amount of fructose in fruits is significantly lower than what's in the sodas and sweets that currently make up the typical modern diet. For example, a serving of strawberries contains a total of 7 grams of sugar, whereas a 16-ounce bottle of soda contains 52 grams! You would have to eat more than 8 cups of strawberries to ingest the equivalent amount of sugar contained in one bottle of soda. A diet high in *whole* fruits and, of course, vegetables has been proven to positively influence our health and well-being. In fact, studies show eight or more servings of fruit and vegetables a day leads to a 30 percent decrease in heart attack and stroke. Specifically, two reviews in the journals *Neurology* and the *Journal of Nutrition* reported that every extra cup serving over the U.S. Department of Agriculture (USDA)–recommended 2 cups per day decreases the risk of stroke by 11 percent and heart disease by 7 percent.

Bottom line: Combining healthy eating habits and exercising on a daily basis with avoidance of added sugar will not only contribute to having the body you have always wanted but also increase the length of your life. Simply put: Ditch the added sugar and you'll probably live a longer, better life.

Low-Carb Diets

As I mentioned, most days I consume no more than 50 grams of carbohydrate. On my low-carb diet I have seen incredible changes not only to my body but also to my mood and concentration. Plus I noticed an enormous increase of my energy level. If you have been struggling with losing weight, cutting carbs is one of the simplest and most effective means at your disposal. Studies show that people on low-carb diets lose more weight, faster, than people on low-fat diets (which are typically high in carbs) . . . even when the low-fat dieters are actively restricting calories.

As for the low-carb vs. low-fat diets, a study conducted over six months reported greater improvements in body composition, insulin sensitivity, and triglycerides in the low-carb group. Although both groups showed improvements in these factors, the most weight was lost in the low-carb group. One of the reasons for this is that low-carb diets tend to get rid of excess water from the body. In response to lower insulin levels, the kidneys start shedding excess sodium, leading to rapid weight loss in the first week or two. The anti-inflammatory benefits of low-carb diets are also beneficial for your overall health.

The real reason low-carb diets work so well, though, is that they remove a lot of processed junk from the diet that tends not to be replaced. Processed foods are cheap and convenient, and generally terrible for you. They grew popular in part because they can last a very long time without spoiling. In fact, I'm sure products like Top Ramen and Twinkies have a half-life that rivals that of radioactive waste. Unfortunately, these are not necessarily good things. Convenience and a long shelf life shouldn't be the determining factors for what enters your stomach.

What's the Deal with Processed Foods?

Almost all prepackaged food sold in cafés and restaurants are loaded with sodium and other preservatives. Transportation and shelf life are two big reasons why. Sodium, alongside other ingredients that sound like chemicals, prevents food products from spoiling as quickly as natural, wholesome foods. This gives them a longer shelf life.

Limit the food you eat in restaurants. Refocus on cooking and preparing meals at home. These two steps can help you avoid the avalanche of sodium and artificial ingredients in much of the standard American diet. Try planning ahead and preparing meals on the weekend if you're facing a busy week.

Water Works

So we've talked about what you should eat. How about drink? Considering our bodies are made up of mostly water, the majority of us know that proper hydration is essential for our well-being. The newborn coming down the Slip 'N Slide of life is 75 percent water. Even as adults we are still 60 percent water, although that percentage decreases as we age. H_2O is the major contributor to human tissue mass in the form of blood plasma and intercellular and interstitial fluids.

Along with water's structural role in the human body, it's integral to a series of critical body functions, including regulation of core temperature, the proper functioning of the kidneys, and the inner workings of the brain. Water lubricates our joints and benefits human metabolism by playing a significant role in digestion. Proper hydration also helps you feel energized. It's important to note that muscles store more water than fat. In fact, muscle cells are considered "wet," whereas fat cells are considered "dry." The more muscle you have, the more necessary it becomes to drink enough water and other fluids.

When the body is dehydrated, it function less well and more slowly. You begin to feel sluggish and lack energy, which affects your day-to-day routines and workouts. You may even experience headaches or even back pain due to dehydration. Dry mouth and thirst are the most obvious signals that you need to drink up. Unfortunately, with our busy lives, we often miss these signals. And guess what? The human body is dehydrated well before thirst kicks in. That's a lagging indicator, not a leading one.

How much fluid do you need? It's simple: Take your weight in pounds, divide by 2, and drink that amount of water in ounces each day as your baseline. For example, if you weigh 120 pounds, drink 60 ounces of fluid daily, most of it water. The human body is made mostly of water . . . not soda. Of course, when working out, you need to drink more. The more you sweat, the more water you should be drinking. Also, make sure to take in fluids one to two hours before your workout. Waiting to drink water right before the session begins may not give your body enough time to become fully hydrated.

Replacing your electrolytes is also important when working out. Electrolytes, such as sodium and potassium, are essential for proper bodily function. When we sweat, we lose electrolytes. Some consider sports drinks like Gatorade to be suitable for electrolyte replacement, though the calories and sugar contained in these drinks leave a lot to be desired. One simple method is to add about ½ teaspoon of sea salt to 1 liter of water and drink it during and after your workout. Or, if you don't love the taste of salty water, I've also known people who simply eat a salt packet—like you'd get at a fast-food joint or diner—then chase it with a few gulps of water. Either way works to get some salt into your system.

Maintaining proper hydration often requires a conscious effort. As with other aspects of well-being and fitness, consistency is key!

Be Wary of Celebrity Diets!

Recently I listened to a hilarious and thoughtful interview with Rebecca Harrington, author of the book *I'll Have What She's Having*. In the book, Harrington examines and explores a bunch of celebrity diets and actually tries them all.

Many of the diets border on the absurd, while others require a top chef to be considered palatable. For example, the Five Hands diet championed by Victoria Beckham allows only five small handfuls of food—usually nuts or some lean protein—a day. The fashion designer Karl Lagerfeld insists on drinking only Diet Coke with an odd nightcap of roasted quail. Sounds practical to me.

Some of the diets actually involve thoughtful planning and execution, but they are also expensive and tedious. Gwyneth Paltrow's diet, though effective, costs, on average, $200 a week. For many that's an entire month's worth of groceries for the whole family! The successful diets followed by Beyoncé and Madonna were so strict, they bordered on torture. Who's going to follow those diets for any length of time?

Don't fall for fad diets. Sure, they may slim you down for a period of time, but you won't stick with them forever, and most of them are no fun. You don't need a fancy way of starving yourself. You need to eat healthy foods, not avoid them!

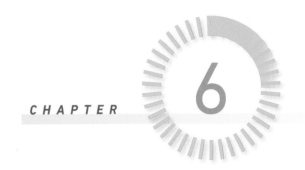

CHAPTER 6

Food Shopping, Appliances, Gadgets, and Cookware

S weat drips down your face. You've been breathing heavily for the past five minutes. Your arms are aching. Your legs are shaking. "How can this be so hard?" you think, realizing it's been a few years since you've done this. How are you sore already? As you stand in front of the open refrigerator, staring at the arsenal of guilt-filled treats, your whole body is telling you one thing: *Stop!*

You've decided to swap out your soda bottles for water bottles, cupcakes for carrots, and mixed nuts for avocados. Well, your mind has. Your belly is waging war on your emotions. Who was there for you when that guy broke your heart? Chocolate cake was. When your boss yelled at you, cookie dough ice cream held you tight all night long. Now ten minutes have lapsed since you opened the refrigerator door; only five minutes remain. Time to rip off the bandage. You chuck everything that has more ingredients than you do fingers, and suddenly the garbage can is full.

Just two minutes left. You still have a stash of chocolate-drizzled cookies in the pantry, so you run to the door and fling it open. You forgot about the box you keep in the nightstand, so you retrieve it and run back to the kitchen, boxes of cookies in hands. You pull the blender out of the cabinet and dump in every cookie, when in walks your boyfriend. "Oh, you're off to a great start!" he says. "What flavor is that protein shake you're making?" To which you respond . . . "Chocolate."

Fitness, here you come.

Your Guide to Grocery Shopping

That example was fictionalized and exaggerated, but you won't clean up your diet until you clean up your fridge. First I want you to pull out a large trash bag. Open it up—you have work to do. Start in the pantry with some of the obvious: cookies, chips, candy, cake mixes, and other snack foods. Say good-bye to Little Debbie and Betty Crocker. Grab them one by one and drop them in the trash bag.

Now it's time to move to the fridge, where the heavy lifting occurs. Grab those metallic sugar bombs by the can or six-pack and drop them in the bag. The same goes for fruit juices and sweetened teas, which are full of added sugar. Even yogurt needs to go, unless it's plain and unsweetened. Otherwise, it too is a source of stealth sugar. Fatty, sodium-laden deli meats and hot dogs are also unhealthy, so pull them off the shelf, along with salad dressings, dipping sauces, and condiments like ketchup and mayonnaise, which are sweetened with corn syrup. See any beer cans or bottles? Yep, those go too.

Close the fridge door and open the freezer. Any ice cream you see needs to be tossed too. Ah, and what are those? Frozen French fries? You don't even need to ask.

Now that I've told you what to toss, you need to know what to fill your kitchen with. So let's go grocery shopping. Most people think they know how to shop in the grocery store, but often they are picking up the wrong items, perhaps without even knowing their mistakes. I'll show you what to look for and what to avoid. When we're done, you'll have all the ingredients you need to make 30 recipes, along with other incidental items.

You should be purchasing about 21 basic items on a weekly basis (see the grocery list on page 68). They can be reconfigured into different recipes, but the ingredients don't need to change very much week to week. Once you grow familiar with your favorite foods and learn the amount of calories each contains, you'll always be able to approximate the number of calories in the meals you make with those ingredients. I'm lucky: The foods that delight my palate also happen to be highly nutritious items such as eggs, nuts, seeds, avocados, apples, oranges, celery, extra-virgin olive oil, and coconut oil. These are among the healthiest foods on the planet, in my opinion. Rich in vital nutrients, they can help you train better, live healthier, and recover from workouts faster, especially the short-burst workouts that constitute this plan.

Healthy food shopping begins long before you ever become captain of your grocery cart. I recommend you make a list before leaving home, based on the recipes you'll find in the pages to come. This will help you get in and out of the store quickly, without having to go down every aisle, especially the cookie aisle. We don't want you to have to check that list twice. Stay away from the cookies, or you'll start to look like Santa. Grocery stores aren't in the nutrition business; they're in the sales business, and their enticing displays are designed to seduce you by appealing to your sense of vision, taste, smell, and texture. When you have your list in hand, sticking with the game plan becomes much easier, even when temptation plays with your emotions. And it will. Are those red velvet brownies? Oops, I mean . . .

I also want you to eat something nutritious before leaving for the market, even if it's just one of the snacks in Chapter 7, or an apple, for that matter. When you're starving as you make your way through the store, *everything* will look delicious. Suddenly, you're making excuses for the food items. "Yeah, it has 31 grams of sugar per serving, but there are 2 grams protein . . . 2 whole grams of protein. That's 2 more grams than cardboard has." Items will practically leap into your cart. In the checkout line, you'll be thinking, "Whoa, how did that bag of Doritos get in my cart? And where did those four jars of Nutella come from, anyway?" The clerk will already be ringing up these "unintentional" purchases by this point. Sheepishly, you'll hand over your credit card and pay for it all. All those unnecessary calories might as well go straight to your hips because we both know you're not going to throw away those items after purchasing them.

Your 21-Item Grocery List!

These superfoods are foods that are particularly rich in macronutrients, micronutrients, and phytonutrients. Many of them are also relatively low in calories and high in fiber. I try to build my diet around these superfoods for the following reasons:

1. It gives me a handy list for grocery shopping and guides my food selection.
2. It's easy to remember the nutrition facts of the most common ingredients I buy on a weekly basis; therefore, I don't need to fall into the trap of counting calories and it works great with my portion-sizing method.
3. It keeps me on track with my healthy lifestyle, providing an affirmative nutrition plan—one that is based around what I should eat rather than focused on what I shouldn't eat.

So without further ado, my 21 favorite superfoods!

Proteins
1. Red meat
2. Salmon
3. Omega-3 eggs
4. Chicken
5. Protein supplements (Vita-Whey, hemp protein, chickpea protein)

Vegetables and Fruits
6. Green leafy vegetables (spinach, kale, collard)
7. Cruciferous vegetables (broccoli, cabbage, cauliflower, Brussels sprouts, bok choy)
8. Low GI fruit and vegetables (berries, oranges, kiwis, peaches, apricots, pears, apples, grapefruits, bell peppers, cucumbers, tomatoes, squash, pumpkin)
9. Root vegetables (carrots, ginger, sweet potatoes)
10. Bulb and stem vegetables (onions, leeks, garlic, celery, asparagus)

Other Carbohydrates

11. Beans and legumes

12. Quinoa

13. Whole oats

Good Fats

14. Nuts and seeds

15. Avocados

16. Extra-virgin olive oil

17. Fish oil

18. Coconut oil and coconut milk

Drinks

19. Green tea

20. Coffee

21. Water

Arrive at the market on a full stomach, or at least with some food in your belly, and better choices become far more likely. The first place to steer your cart is the produce section, which lies on the perimeter of most markets. That's where you'll find most of the healthy foods because that is where ventilation, refrigeration, and water are located. No need for such conditions for row after row of breakfast cereals and cookies. So all the junk ends up in the middle aisles.

To me the produce section is the most exciting part of the supermarket; I love the beautiful rainbow of colors on display and the plethora of fresh smells. It's like Mother Nature's version of *Charlie and the Chocolate Factory*. Unlike a candy store, where the colors sugarcoat harmful substances, the colors in the produce section reflect the diverse array of vitamins, minerals, and phytonutrients in those foods. Carotenoids impart the yellow and orange colors. Greens look that way because they contain chlorophyll; blue and red produce have a high concentration of flavonoids. All these compounds help explain why fruit and vegetables have a strong association with a reduced risk for numerous diseases. For whatever reason, these compounds seem to work better together than alone. As a result, it's better to eat a variety of fruits and vegetables than it is to take any one of their nutrients in concentrated form, as you would find in, say, the supplement form of a single antioxidant such as vitamin C.

The first things I want you to look for in this section are spinach and broccoli, which are staples in my kitchen. We're turning you into the Green Giant. Highly nutritious, low-calorie foods, they lavish your body with fiber, vitamins, antioxidants, and minerals. Both of these vegetables are also yummy and versatile. I make salads from spinach all the time, especially for lunch or dinner, often pairing it with salmon. If you have no clue what to eat at a given moment, think broccoli and spinach, not chocolate cake and French fries. Scrambling eggs with steamed broccoli makes for a delicious and healthy breakfast, one that starts your day off on the right foot. You will feel satisfied and energized, not stuffed and weighed down or bloated.

Fruit, not ice cream and candy bars, should be your source of sugar. Like veggies, fruits are found in the produce section on the perimeter of the supermarket or grocery store. Berries, apples, pears, kiwis, grapefruits, tangerines, oranges, cherries, peaches, and apricots—I love fruit! Pick up several different kinds every time you food shop, but on your first trip, I insist that you pick up some blueberries! These flavonoid-rich fruits should be a staple of everyone's daily diet. They support cognitive and motor function while preventing many diseases. Blueberries also have been shown to improve muscle recovery after an intense workout, a huge help on this program. The better and faster the recovery from working out, the greater the progress will be in your body composition, energy, strength and overall fitness.

The positive effects of blueberries extend to the brain. If you forget to eat your blueberries, you'll eventually forget all kinds of other stuff too. Memory loss often comes with age, but it can also be triggered and aggravated by stress, anxiety, and depression. A diet with ample blueberries may help reduce all of those symptoms.

Owing to their low glycemic index value and high fiber quotient, blueberries are also great for regulating blood sugar levels. Even if you have metabolic syndrome or insulin resistance, blueberries can help keep your blood sugar from drifting up to the levels diagnostic of prediabetes (fasting blood glucose from 100 milligrams per deciliter to 125 milligrams per deciliter) or type 2 diabetes (fasting blood glucose equal to or greater than 126 milligrams per deciliter). Your cardiovascular system, which can be preserved or harmed by your glucose metabolism, depending on how well it works, will also benefit if you start eating blueberries daily. The good news is that you can freeze fresh blueberries with no loss of health benefits. They will keep the same levels of antioxidants, vitamins, and fiber, and they make a great addition to your postworkout smoothies.

I mentioned eggs earlier in the book, and that should be your next acquisition in the supermarket. Usually eggs are found on the perimeter of the store along with the dairy. I love eggs, and their nutrition profile is excellent. A single egg has 75 calories, and along with those calories come 7 grams of protein and 5 grams of fat, not to mention numerous vitamins and minerals. Eggs are particularly rich in lutein and zeaxanthin, two carotenoids that help prevent eye diseases, such as cataracts and macular degeneration.

Not only are eggs supernutritious but they are also incredibly versatile. They can be scrambled, poached, hard-boiled, or prepared any number of other ways. You can turn them into omelets or frittatas that also include healthy vegetables. Eggs are particularly great for breakfast because their macronutrient profile makes them more satiating than cereal-based breakfasts, muffins, and the like. Eggs for breakfast means less chance of overeating later in the day.

Chicken is another great protein source. In fitness circles, chicken is synonymous with bodybuilders, who scarf it down during contest season because it's lower in fat, less expensive, and easier to cook than red meat. Fat is an issue for them because they are aiming for single-digit body fat on contest day. I don't recommend eating chicken constantly like they do, but it works great as an entrée, in a Crock-Pot, or on top of a salad.

I also eat quite a bit of fish, especially salmon and tuna. Dietary omega-3 polyunsaturated fatty acids (PUFAs) appear to play an important in the prevention of both cognitive decline and diseases such as prostate cancer, depression, stroke, and cardiovascular disease, particularly sudden cardiac death. Note that *how* the fish (and other foods) is prepared is very important! A study by the American Heart Association published in *Circulation* reported that consuming broiled or baked tuna, salmon, mahimahi, and other fish reduced the risk of developing cardiovascular risk factors compared to individuals who ate the same fish but fried. The same study indicated that consuming fish or foods rich in omega-3 fatty acids three or more times a week was more beneficial than eating them less than once a week, with the minimum recommendation of *at least* once a week.

Last, pick up some hemp protein. If you're making a salad and you don't want to use meat as your protein source, sprinkle the hemp protein over it to add protein.

As I move my cart through the aisles, I'm also on the lookout for healthy fats. So I pick up an avocado, which is actually a fruit—bet you didn't know that. I also grab a bottle of extra-virgin olive oil. Nuts and seeds are another great snack, and ones that usually contain healthy fats. I like to use coconut products, such as coconut oil and coconut milk, as another source of good fats. I don't avoid dairy products such as butter, cheese, or heavy cream, either—as long as it's grass-fed and non-GMO.

Raise a Glass to Your Health

For drinks, I'm a big believer in water, tea, and coffee. You don't necessarily need to get your water at the supermarket, so let's focus on green tea, probably the closest

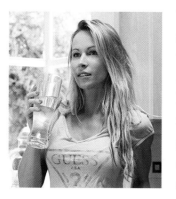

thing we have to a health elixir. A big reason is that green tea contains catechins, which are antioxidants that protect the cells in your body against damage. Studies find that green tea improves blood flow and lowers cholesterol. This is a boon to cardiovascular, metabolic, and brain health. Epigallocatechin-3-gallate (EGCG) is the most powerful and abundant catechin contained in green tea and is the most available to be absorbed by the body once it is digested.

According to a study in the *British Journal of Nutrition*, green tea catechins also protect against cancer cell proliferation, insulin resistance, and accelerated aging. Now who wouldn't want that? I drink at least one cup of tea daily. I don't add sugar to it. Neither should you. You're sweet enough already.

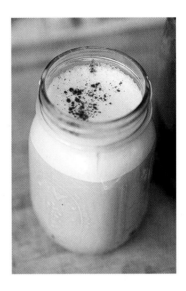

I also love a good cup of coffee. This beverage was once suspected of being a vice—anything this good must be unhealthy, right? Yet a growing body of evidence suggests that your body benefits from a few cups of coffee a day. These benefits include a reduction in your risk for type 2 diabetes, liver disease, and cardiovascular disease.

Population studies have established that the body responds to coffee in complicated ways. For starters, coffee consumption increases circulating cholesterol. This can be considered a good or a bad thing, depending on what the body does with the circulating cholesterol. The bad is that the cholesterol can be redeposited in the blood vessels and contribute to plaque buildup. The good? The circulating cholesterol can be used as an energy source, so instead of using glucose or muscle glycogen as your workout fuel, you burn fats! Coffee also has similar antioxidant properties to those found in green tea.

Of course, at the risk of stating the obvious, coffee also gives you that little extra somethin'-somethin' for your workouts, and the better your workouts, the fitter and healthier you'll become. I'll drink to that. As is true of green tea, all this good news evaporates if you ruin a perfectly good cup of coffee by pouring a bunch of sugar into it. Yuck.

Beware of Health Food Impostors

As I mentioned earlier in this chapter, supermarkets are retailers. They just happen to be selling food. Manufacturers know that a certain segment of their customer base has been conditioned to look for healthy fare. So many products are marketed for their health benefits. Unfortunately, many of these products are *not* healthy. One notable example from a few years ago was the claim by General Mills that Cheerios were heart healthy because they lack saturated fat and cholesterol. First, it's become apparent that saturated fat and dietary cholesterol don't have all that much to do with cholesterol levels or heart disease. Second, Cheerios are really just a big carb load made even bigger when poured into a bowl of milk, which contains lactose, a natural form of sugar. In 2009 General Mills received a letter from the FDA asking it to change its marketing tactics for Cheerios on account of "unauthorized health claims."

Supermarkets are full of fake health foods like Cheerios. I can't warn you about all of them, but a few deserve special attention, starting with yogurt. The majority of sales are for yogurt that has been sweetened with added sugars, which is not a health food. A gut bomb with probiotics is still a gut bomb. I even stopped buying Greek yogurt because it's often full of sugar. I switched to sour cream, which has more calories, so I stick to small portions.

Nothing equals the confusion surrounding whole-grain bread and similar products, though. Many people now know that white bread is not good for you. Great. Beyond that, however, most people would tell you any bread product with the words "wheat" or "grain" on the wrapper is a health food. However, while most of these products look more or less the same, many of them are not exactly healthy, which is one reason why my list of recipes has no sandwiches. When was the last time you saw a fit person eating a sandwich, anyway? Seriously, think about that for a moment. Fit people realize that healthy foods don't need to be squeezed between two pieces of bread to taste good. And they don't want those extra carbs either.

If you don't want to skip bread altogether, let me at least offer some guidance on the confusing terminology. A kernel of grain is made up of three parts: the bran, the endosperm, and the germ. Whole grain contains them all. Whole wheat loses the bran and germ in the refining process, leaving only the endosperm. Most of the healthy nutrients such as vitamin B, not to mention the fiber, reside in the bran and germ. So whole wheat bread isn't much better than white bread. If you're still inclined to buy bread, look for "whole wheat flour" as the first ingredient on the label or the phrase *100% whole grain*. If you see either of those, go for it.

Alternatively, simply bake your own nutritious bread. I have two different recipes for you in this book.

You just can't go wrong with this grocery list. You can be really creative. You can add any herbs you like (see "Little-Known Ways to Make Clean Food Taste Amazing" below), and you can make juices or smoothies if you don't like to eat salads too often. The options are endless. Once you see results and notice the awesome feeling that eating healthfully brings, you won't turn back!

Little-Known Ways to Make Clean Food Taste Amazing

For lots of people, healthy eating conjures up images of bland, tasteless rabbit food, but that isn't the way it has to be. Here are some very simple ways to make healthy food irresistible!

The Magic of Herbs and Spices!

Herbs and spices don't have much of an impact on your caloric intake, but they have a *huge* impact on taste. Even if you don't always have fresh herbs on hand, dried herbs and ground spices in a well-stocked spice cabinet are an excellent substitute. Rosemary, ginger, sage, and thyme, to name just a few, will bring your foods to life, and half the fun is discovering the flavor combinations you like best. Try fresh lime, fresh cilantro, and dried red pepper flakes for Mexican-inspired meats, soups, fish, and vegetables. Take a chicken breast from blah to *wow* with fresh or dried rosemary, and fall in love with veggies by highlighting their natural flavor with sea salt, fresh garlic, and your favorite spices. With a little experimenting, you will find the possibilities are endless!

Get Roasting!

Let's face it, there's only so much steamed broccoli you can handle before you're ready to throw in the towel. Roasting veggies in the oven using high heat, 400 to 450°F, concentrates their flavor and brings out their mild sweetness as their natural sugars

(continues)

caramelize. Vegetables like Brussels sprouts and cauliflower, which you may never have liked in the past, take on a whole different flavor profile when roasted, and the process couldn't be easier. Chop the veggies down to a uniform size if needed, toss them with a very light coating of the oil of your choice and a sprinkling of coarse salt, then roast until soft and browned to your liking. Before serving, toss them with some fresh herbs and a dash of freshly squeezed lemon juice or Parmesan cheese . . . so easy and so delicious!

Get a Little Nutty!

Freshly roasted nuts add texture, taste, and richness to almost any meal. Pine nuts are a perfect complement to sautéed spinach, broccoli rabe, and other sautéed greens. Toasted walnuts are naturals on salad, oatmeal, rice, or couscous. Slivered almonds or pecans are amazing on fruits, chicken, and fish. To toast: Spread the nuts on a rimmed baking sheet and heat in a 250°F oven for 4 to 6 minutes, watching carefully to ensure that they don't burn. A 2-tablespoon serving adds only about 90 calories, and they are a great source of healthy fats!

Stocking Your Kitchen

Once those delicious and healthy foods fill your cupboards and fridge, you'll need appliances, gadgets, and cookware to prepare your meals. None of this stuff is terribly expensive, and the money you'll save by not eating out as much will more than cover the cost. And what price can you put on your health?

1. Nonstick Pots and Pans

Nonstick pots and pans in a variety of sizes are the perfect way to cook delicious, healthful foods without adding calories from added fats! Cutting down on your use of added fats in your daily cooking can save you hundreds of calories.

2. Basic Utensils

Every great kitchen starts with the basics, and every job needs the right tool. Make sure to get a silicone spatula, a four-ounce ladle, tongs, a whisk, a couple of wooden spoons, and rubber or silicone scrapers. These handy gadgets, along with your knives and cutting boards, will help you on your way to culinary greatness!

3. Mixing Bowls

The uses for mixing bowls are endless, and they are crucial for bringing amazing flavor to your dinner table! Experiment with different spices, herbs, vinegars, and healthy oils to create marinades for chicken or dressings for salads.

4. Cutting Boards and a Basic Knife Set

When it comes to food prep, you really need only three quality knives to get cooking: an 8-inch chef's knife, a paring knife, and a bread knife. There really isn't anything you can't tackle with those kitchen classics. Also, be sure to have a variety of sturdy cutting boards, especially one you use only for raw meat.

5. Can Opener

Even the healthiest of eaters needs to open a can sometimes, so it's good to have a can opener that works while being safe at the same time. Look for one that opens the can while leaving the top intact with a smooth edge.

6. Measuring Cups and Spoons

Measuring cups and spoons are additional kitchen necessities that serve double duty. Not only will they ensure that your recipes come out perfect every time, but they are also a great way to know exactly how many calories you're adding to your meals.

7. Colanders and Strainers

Colanders are good for a lot more than just draining pasta! You can wash and store fruits and vegetables in them, and a metal colander can even be used as a steamer! Strainers have a fine mesh, which make them perfect for straining delicious broths.

8. Six-Sided Grater and Peeler

A six-sided grater is like a Swiss Army Knife for your kitchen. Extra-fine, coarse, and even julienne options means there's nothing you can't handle. Be sure to have a comfortable, sturdy peeler in your drawer as well!

9. Potato Masher

Potato mashers aren't just for potatoes! Use yours to make easy work of egg salad, guacamole, stewed tomatoes, and even crushing nuts! It also makes a good tool for breaking up ground meat while it's browning.

10. Silicone Basting Brush

A basting brush is an absolute must-have for adding flavor and moisture to meats, especially during the cooking process. For a basting brush, silicone is your best bet; it's not only heat resistant but also easy to clean and stain- and odor-resistant.

11. Blender and Juicer

Never pay outrageous sums for a smoothie again! Invest in your own blender and juicer, and you'll be able to make all of your favorite smoothie recipes right in your own kitchen, any time day or night. I rely on my Vitamix blender a lot. Yes, it's expensive, but it has a lifetime guarantee, and I can't afford to buy cheap blenders that break or don't do their job.

12. Baking Sheets

Baking sheets are good for a lot more than just baking cookies. You can use them to perfectly roast your favorite vegetables, bake chicken breasts, and even toast your favorite nuts to enhance your favorite recipes.

13. Cupcake and Muffin Pans

Muffin pans aren't just for carb-loaded cupcakes. You can make your own mini egg breakfast quiches or delicious protein muffins and freeze them for easy, on-the-go snacks. Choose nonstick for super-easy cleanup.

14. Baking Dishes

A few basic baking dishes will carry you a long way. A 9-by-13-inch glass baking dish will always be put to good use, and an 8-inch loaf pan and an 8-inch square baking pan will serve you well too. You can choose from glass, ceramic, or metal.

15. Kitchen Towels and Oven Mitts

No matter how strong and tough you are, you're going to need quality oven mitts. Look for ones with silicone ribbing, which provide a secure grip when you are removing hot pans from the oven. To keep your kitchen clean, washable kitchen towels will be an indispensable addition to your culinary toolbox.

16. Storage Containers

Always be sure to have a wide variety of storage containers with lids ready and waiting. They are perfect for leftovers and for portioning out your meals. Whether you prefer glass or plastic, there are tons of sizes available to suit your needs.

17. Steamer

An important part of any healthy diet is lots of veggies, and steaming is a great way to cook your vegetables while retaining their nutritional benefits. You can choose a stovetop steamer or an electric one. As an added bonus, electric steamers can also cook rice as well as hard-boil eggs.

Five Powerful Vegetables You May Not Know About

A recent study categorized 47 different fruits and vegetables based on the number of important nutrients each food contained. Each fruit or vegetable was classified based on the level of 17 specific nutrients considered vital for health and for the prevention of chronic diseases according to international standards. A score was assigned to each fruit or vegetable according to the level of these essential nutrients—100 being the highest and, of course, 0 being the lowest. Foods with the highest scores were defined as powerhouse fruits and vegetables (PFVs).

The results were quite surprising. Here are the top five. Some were new to me. Enjoy!

1. **Watercress:** This scored a perfect 100 as a PFV! Apparently, it is one of the very first plants consumed by early humans, and today it's used often in Europe and Asia. Watercress packs a surprising punch when it comes to vitamin C levels.
2. **Chinese cabbage:** Often used in Asian cuisine, this is high in vitamins A and C.
3. **Chard:** This doppelgänger for lettuce may not have the most appetizing name, but it's used quite a bit in Mediterranean cooking, especially in salads. Chard is rich in minerals and high in vitamins A, C, and K.
4. **Beet greens:** More nutrient-dense than beets themselves, beet greens also work well in salads and are astonishingly high in vitamin A.
5. **Spinach:** Finally! A vegetable that we all know and love! Spinach has always been a perennial powerhouse when it comes to nutrients. It scored an 86 in the study. Spinach is especially high in iron as well as other minerals and vitamins.

Should You Be Taking Dietary Supplements?

When it comes to supplements, I take them at their name—supplements. I don't look at them as magic substances that will make me stronger, better, faster, slimmer, or sexier. They are a convenient way to get the nutrients my body needs, when real food is unavailable.

Nutritional supplements fall into two major categories: *essential nutrients* and *nonessential nutrients*.

Essential Nutrients

Essential nutrients are those that we need for normal physiological functioning and that are present in food. These nutrients must be digested because the body doesn't have the capacity to make them itself.

Although no supplements are absolutely essential, a low intake of calories, macronutrients, or micronutrients is common due to our busy lifestyles. For bad days and times when food is not readily available, the following three staple supplements are always good to keep on hand:

1. **Protein supplement:** The one I use most commonly is flavorless.
   Food equivalent: any complete protein source, including meat, fish, poultry, egg whites.
2. **Greens supplement:** These are full of antioxidants.
   Food equivalent: vegetables, fruit.
3. **Fish oil supplement:** These offer a host of health benefits.
   Food equivalent: salmon, anchovy, sardine, flaxseeds, chia seeds, enriched eggs, grass-fed beef, walnuts.

Nonessential Nutrients

Nonessential nutrients are food-based nutrients that your body can make itself, or nutrients that aren't needed for normal physiological functioning. While they're obviously not on the top of the nutritional priority list, they're still very popular

(continues)

because some of them produce positive benefits when used specifically to enhance certain physiological responses. Here are two examples of nonessential nutrient supplements:

1. **Caffeine:** before your workout to improve central nervous system output.
2. **Green tea extract:** daily during times when you're actively trying to lose weight to stimulate metabolism.

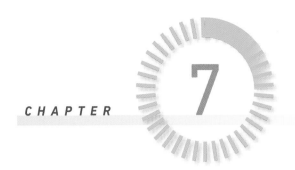
Recipes for Success

Diet is something that people struggle with way more than even some of my most intense workout routines. To some, picking up an apple as opposed to a fork for a big ol' slab of cake is harder than doing 30 burpees. I have a theory regarding this phenomenon. I can tell you exactly what workout to do every day, and you can just do it. In contrast, I am not there each time you're supposed to eat. Instead of me making the choices and plans for you, your hungry, reckless stomach is calling the shots. Maybe one day I will have a smartphone app that will allow me to yell at you each time you skip your breakfast or stop you with a little electric shock each time you try to binge. Unfortunately, that app has not been developed yet. (In progress: to be released spring 2020.)

I'm kidding, of course, but diets can truly be harder to follow than workout plans. Which is why I'm not really giving you a diet per se. "Diets" have a beginning and an end by definition, whereas I'm teaching you how to eat healthfully for the rest of your life. This is much more consistent with the Greek meaning for the word *diet*: "a way of eating." When they weren't inventing democracy or sculpting statues, the ancient Greeks took a holistic view of nutrition, making it central to a healthy lifestyle, although they wouldn't have called it that. I'm sure if they saw some of the crazy diets practiced today, lacking basic nutrition in some cases, they would roll over in their graves.

So you now understand the basics of clean eating as well as my nutritional philosophy. You've cleaned out the fridge and shopped for healthier fare. You have all the kitchen tools you need at your disposal. You are ready to go. In this chapter you'll find 30 delicious recipes for healthy breakfasts, lunches, dinners, snacks, smoothies, and juices to keep you fueled for your workouts and energized for your day. Healthy eating doesn't take a ton of time; most of the recipes I provide in this chapter can be prepared in no more than 15 minutes.

Portions over Calories

Counting calories is unnecessary for many people, in my opinion. I'd rather pay attention to my portion sizes. This gives me an easier way to measure the right amount of food I eat on a daily basis. That being said, counting calories can be the next step if portion sizes fail to help you reach your goal. Let me give you an example: A 30-year-old woman who has always been skinny—let's call her Zelda—wants to put on muscle. She might say something like "I can't put on any weight even though I eat a lot." Several acquaintances of mine fit Zelda's description, and they all share at least two things in common:

1. They feel like they eat a lot.

2. They actually don't eat enough.

First, identify your activity level from among these:

1. **Sedentary:** minimal exercise, maybe yoga or aerobic exercise; mostly sitting at work.

2. **Moderately active:** sedentary job, but following a daily workout schedule.

3. **Very active:** following my program plus doing a lot of sports and activities, having an active job, basically moving all day long and doing high-intensity workouts regularly.

Once you figure out your activity level, calculate how many calories a day you should be eating based on your goal. Here's an easy-to-use calorie estimator:

Your Activity Level	Your Goal Is Weight Loss	Your Goal Is Weight Maintenance	Your Goal Is Weight Gain
	Multiply your body weight in pounds by:		
Sedentary	10 to 12	12 to 14	16 to 18
Moderately Active	12 to 14	14 to 16	18 to 20
Very Active	14 to 16	16 to 18	20 to 22

To demonstrate how this works in practice, let's have a look at a couple of examples.

Example 1

A 150-pound, moderately active reader interested in fat loss would begin by taking in between 1,800 (150 × 12) and 2,100 (150 × 14) calories a day.

Example 2

A 120-pound very active reader interested in muscle gain would start by taking in between 2,400 (120 × 20) and 2,640 (120 × 22) calories a day.

Factoring in Meal Frequency

I recommend eating every three to four hours. Only during the day, though—I don't want you waking up at night. Your digestive system needs to rest overnight. What's more, interrupted sleep will cause hormonal disruptions that favor weight gain rather than loss. Finally, you may sleep with someone, and I pity them if you're getting up at all hours of the night to eat.

To stay on track with my meals, I set the alarm on my smartphone. I recommend this to anyone who tends to forget about eating and therefore skip meals, which can lead to overeating once he or she realizes, *Hey, I haven't eaten in eight hours!* I have my routine down at this point, but I still like the reminder, just in case I'm in the middle of meetings or doing a video shoot. If you want to make it really easy on yourself, set your alarm to go off four times daily at four-hour intervals. For example, if your first meal is at 8 a.m., your last meal would be at 8 p.m. You also would eat at noon and 4 p.m. Pick your favorite four nutritious meals and eat the same way each day for the entire week. It's easy to keep your calories in check if you know your meals and how many calories you are taking in. You can then change up the meals each week to keep it fresh.

So let's look at how all of this ties together. Let's say you are a woman who weighs 160 pounds and wants to lose weight. Take that number, 160, and multiply it by 12. To accomplish your goals, your daily caloric intake shouldn't exceed 1,920.

Portion Sizes

Earlier I gave you a simple formula for how many calories to consume each day based on your goals. However, not everyone needs or wants to count calories. I don't. Frankly, it's a little bit of a hassle for me, and besides, it's not always accurate. If you rely on searching for nutrition facts in handbooks, websites, or apps, the data you access may or may not be correct. In fact, research has shown they can be off by about 25 percent because of measurement errors, incorrect labeling, or food quality. Your own caloric expenditure comes with another 25 percent margin for error. So it's tough to determine exactly how many calories you burn on any given day, since it varies depending on leisure activities, workouts, and individual differences. The good news is that calorie counting is often unnecessary. The secret is right there in the palm of your hand, with this visual guide to determining portion sizes:

- Your palm determines your protein portions.

- Your cupped hands determine your veggie portions.

- One cupped hand determines your carb and fruit portions.

- Your thumb determines your fat portions.

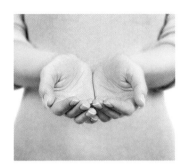

Eating on the Go

Ever have one of those crazy days when you're busy nonstop? Maybe you're constantly on the go; maybe work is out of control, leaving zero time to cook or prepare a single healthy meal. So you buy whatever's available to address the hunger pains, and that's probably not going to be a salad. Perhaps you didn't have much of a choice, but that still makes you feel guilty or frustrated. You want to eat healthfully—and you had been doing so well until today.

I know how that feels, and that's why I plan ahead. Often that means packing meals and keeping healthy snacks—nuts, an apple, homemade granola, and so on—at hand. Admittedly, I may not always end up with something super delicious when I brown-bag it for a busy day, but I always make sure to eat something nutritious, even if it's simple and unadorned. That being said, you may have more culinary skills than I do, in which case, all you need in order to enjoy a healthy and delicious meal is an awesome lunch box you can take with you!

Tracking Your Progress

Do you know how to track your weight loss without driving yourself crazy? I have a friend who is pretty much obsessed with checking her body weight. She steps on the scale *at least* four times a day. She weighs herself in the morning, before she eats, after she eats, and before she goes to bed. I wouldn't be surprised if she has obsessive-compulsive disorder at this point.

Obviously she's not always happy with the results; even the slightest fluctuations can upset her terribly. I've tried to talk her out of this craziness, but some people stubbornly stick with their habits, no matter how useless they are or even how much pain these habits bring them. Can you imagine having your mood rise and fall with the number on a scale? Even worse, imagine having a perfect number in your mind, one you're stuck on, one that you believe is perfect, and it can't be off by even a pound. The only thing that you would be accomplishing at this point is causing yourself tremendous pain.

If you'd ask me how much I weigh, I would say somewhere between 121 to 125 pounds. I don't know exactly, and, to be perfectly honest, I don't even care. The only person that really keeps track of my weight is my doctor, and she notes it only once a year. The truth is that the number on the scale is not as important as you might think. The only time that I would recommend to track your weight biweekly is if you were obese or really overweight and your goal was to get back into the healthy range. There are many women, though, who are in the healthy range, and yet they're still obsessed with what the scale says.

If you're exercising on a regular basis, you're most likely building lean muscle tissue, which is more dense than fat. That means you may be gaining weight on the scale while looking thinner in the mirror. If you know you're not far from your goal, it's helpful to use a measuring tape. A tape is also the best way to keep your problem areas in check, such as your thighs, hips, and love handles.

When you're using the measuring tape, always measure the same area. If you are measuring your thighs, for example, always measure the mid part. You would get very different and confusing results if you measure your waistline one day above your belly button and seven days later below your belly button. Always write down not only the number but also exact part of your body. If you are measuring biceps, thighs, and calves, always wrap the measuring tape around the middle of the muscle. Your waist should be measured just above your belly button, and your hips around your hipbones. Finally, don't obsess too much about keeping track of your measurements. Checking your weight loss progress once a week is more than enough!

Recipes

Flank Steak with Radicchio Salad and Sherry Dressing

Vitamin B_{12} and iron are both very important components of our diet, and it's much easier—and more delicious—to get them from food than from vitamin supplements. Look for grass-fed beef from a local farm, if possible. You can swap radicchio for cabbage—it will be just as delicious.

INGREDIENTS

½ medium red onion, coarsely chopped

5 tablespoons sherry vinegar

4 tablespoons balsamic vinegar

2 garlic cloves, minced

⅔ cup grapeseed oil

1 pound flank steak

Salt and freshly ground pepper to taste

1 medium red bell pepper, coarsely chopped

1 small head radicchio

2 cups mixed greens (arugula, baby spinach)

½ cup crumbled feta cheese

1 small shallot, coarsely chopped

2 tablespoons agave nectar

3 tablespoons extra-virgin olive oil

INSTRUCTIONS

1. Mix the onion with 2 tablespoons of the sherry vinegar, 2 tablespoons of the balsamic vinegar, the garlic, and 2 tablespoons of the grapeseed oil in a medium bowl. Let sit at room temperature for 15 minutes while you prepare the steak.

2. Place the flank steak on a cutting board and with a very sharp knife cut it into very thin strips. Slice against the grain on a slight diagonal (not exactly 90 degrees to the grain). Season generously with salt and pepper.

3. Coat a frying pan with a thin layer of the grapeseed oil and heat over medium-high heat. (The oil should sizzle when you add the steak.) Spread the flank steak into a single layer in the pan (you may have to cook it in batches) and let it cook, without stirring, for about 1 minute, or until golden brown. Then turn and let it cook 30 seconds

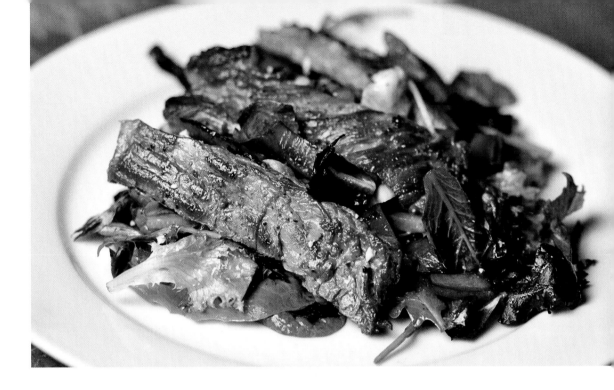

or until golden brown. Remove the meat, place it on a plate, and cover to keep it warm. Repeat the process if you need to cook the steak in batches.

4. Add the onion mixture to the same pan with the leftover oil and juices from the steak. Sauté, stirring occasionally, about 2 minutes or until slightly brown. Add the bell pepper and cook 4 to 6 minutes or until brown. Season with salt and pepper.

5. In the meantime, chop the radicchio and place it in a large bowl; mix in the greens. When the onions and peppers are done, drain them and add them to the radicchio and toss together with the feta cheese and flank steak.

6. Make the dressing: Place the shallot, agave nectar, the remaining 3 tablespoons of sherry vinegar, the remaining 2 tablespoons of balsamic vinegar, the olive oil, and the remaining ¼ cup of grapeseed oil in a blender. Blend on high until well mixed. Season with salt and pepper.

7. Use roughly 2 tablespoons of the dressing over your delicious flank steak radicchio salad.

8. Refrigerate the leftover dressing, which should be good for 3 days.

Quinoa with Cauliflower, Chicken, and Mint Dressing

I love the combination of salty, sweet, and sour flavors in this dish. It makes a great lunch or dinner. If you want to make it a free meal, you can swap the quinoa for roasted broccoli or carrots.

DRESSING

2 tablespoons peanut oil

1 teaspoon agave nectar

1 tablespoon champagne vinegar

¼ cup finely chopped fresh mint

Salt and freshly ground pepper to taste

INGREDIENTS

2 cups water

1 cup cauliflower florets

1 tablespoon grapeseed oil

1 cup chopped skinless boneless chicken thighs

2 tablespoons golden raisins

Salt and freshly ground pepper to taste

½ cup cooked quinoa (multicolor or red)

INSTRUCTIONS

1. Make the dressing: Mix the peanut oil, agave nectar, champagne vinegar, mint, salt, and pepper in a small bowl until well blended.

2. Make the quinoa: Insert a vegetable steamer in a medium saucepan and bring the water to a boil over high heat. When the water starts boiling, reduce the heat to medium and place the cauliflower in the steamer. Cover and let steam until soft, 6 to 10 minutes. Use a fork to check if the cauliflower is tender.

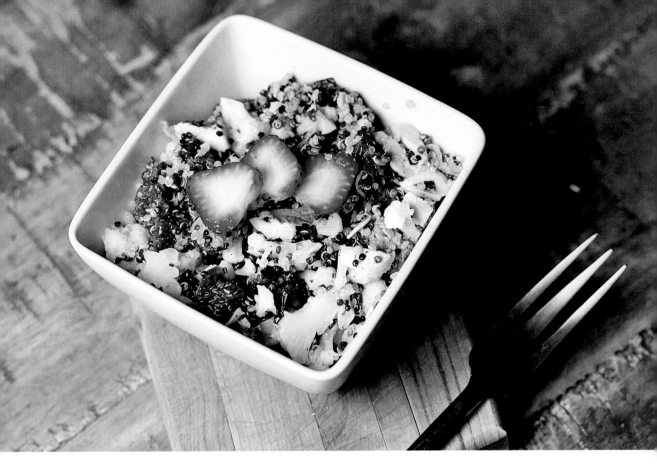

3. Coat a medium frying pan with a thin layer of grapeseed oil and heat over medium-high heat. Add the chicken. (The oil should sizzle when you add the chicken.) Cook the chicken until cooked through, about 15 minutes. Add the raisins to the pan about 2 minutes before the chicken is done. Remove from the heat and season with salt and pepper.

4. Combine the quinoa, chicken mixture, and cauliflower in a large bowl and add a couple of tablespoons of dressing as desired. You can store the rest of the dressing in the fridge for a few days.

> Note: I like to keep my cooked quinoa in the fridge so I can use it in recipes throughout the week.

Steak with Brandy Cream Sauce and Roasted Carrots

I like making this recipe when I have guests over at my house. The sauce is an old French recipe, and the flavor really stands out. Along with being delicious, it's really fun to make because it requires you to ignite the brandy in the skillet. You must be careful, but once you learn how to light it without burning down your kitchen, it'll be one of your favorite meals to cook and serve your friends. You don't have to earn this meal with a workout. It's full of protein, fiber, healthy fats, and the little bit of alcohol in the sauce isn't unhealthy.

INGREDIENTS

4 cups peeled and sliced carrots (2 inches long and ¼ inch thick)

3 tablespoons extra-virgin olive oil

Salt and freshly ground pepper to taste

4 tenderloin steaks (6–8 ounces each and 1½ inches thick)

3 tablespoons avocado oil

1 tablespoon unsalted butter

⅓ cup plus 1 teaspoon brandy

1 cup heavy cream

INSTRUCTIONS

1. Preheat the oven to 400°F. Place the carrot pieces on a large rimmed baking sheet, drizzle with olive oil, and then rub the olive oil into the carrots with your hands. Wash your hands and add salt and pepper. Toss the carrots around in the baking sheet until the salt and pepper evenly coats the carrots.

2. Bake the carrots for 45 to 50 minutes, until you see golden-brown blisters forming on top of the carrot pieces. The carrots should be crunchy on top and soft in the middle.

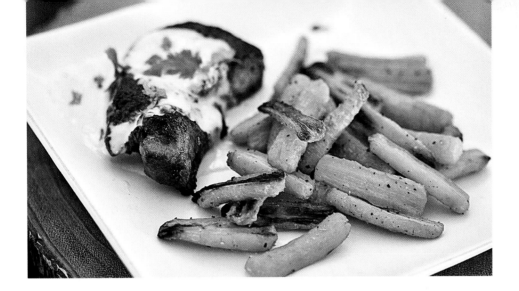

3. While the carrots bake, sprinkle all sides of the steaks generously with salt and pepper. Let the steaks sit on the counter at room temperature for 30 minutes, then heat up the avocado oil and butter in a nonstick skillet over medium heat.

4. When the butter and oil begin to turn golden brown and smoke, gently place the steaks in the skillet. For medium-rare doneness, cook on each side for 4 minutes.

5. Remove the steaks to a plate, cover with foil, and set aside. Turn off the heat and use the same pan with the juices to make the brandy cream sauce.

6. Let the pan cool for about 3 minutes, then pour ⅓ cup of the brandy into the pan. Carefully ignite the alcohol with a long match. Shake the skillet very gently until the flames die.

7. Return the skillet to medium heat and add the cream. Stirring continuously, bring the cream and brandy to a boil until the sauce coats the back of the spoon, about 5 minutes. Add the remaining 1 teaspoon of brandy and season with salt to taste.

8. Add the steaks back to the pan, spoon the sauce over them, and serve with the roasted carrots. The carrots should be done around the same time you finish the steaks and sauce.

Pan-Seared Ahi Tuna with Broccoli and Sweet-and-Sour Avocado Dressing

It's true that searing the tuna just right without overcooking it can be a challenge the first time you try, but once you get that down, this will become one of your favorite dinners to make. It's fresh, delicious, fancy, and fast!

DRESSING

2 tablespoons avocado

1 teaspoon Dijon mustard

1 teaspoon agave nectar

2 tablespoons champagne vinegar

½ cup grapeseed oil

½ small shallot, minced

2 tablespoons freshly squeezed orange juice

INGREDIENTS

2 cups chopped broccoli florets

2 tablespoons extra-virgin olive oil

Salt and freshly ground pepper to taste

Two 5-ounce sushi-quality tuna steaks

2 tablespoons grapeseed oil

¼ cup ricotta salata (or feta cheese)

INSTRUCTIONS

1. Preheat the oven to 400°F.

2. Make the dressing: Place the avocado, mustard, agave nectar, champagne vinegar, grapeseed oil, shallot, and orange juice in a blender. Blend on medium until smooth.

3. Place the broccoli on a large rimmed baking sheet, drizzle with the olive oil to coat, and spread out in a single layer. Season with salt and pepper and roast for 20 to 25 minutes (shake the pan from time to time), until slightly charred. When the broccoli's done, set it aside to cool.

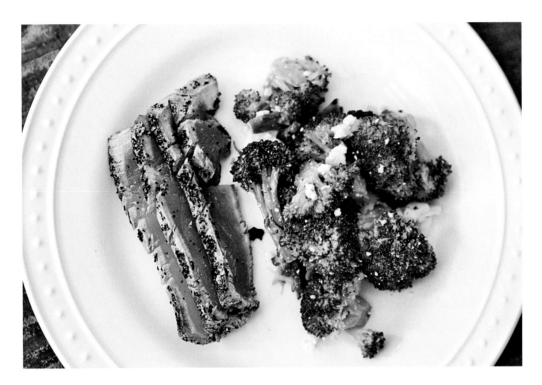

4. Combine about 1 teaspoon of salt and 1 teaspoon of pepper on a small plate and mix with your fingers. Pat the tuna dry with a paper towel and then coat each side evenly with the salt and pepper mixture. The seasoning should be visible on the tuna.

5. Coat a skillet with grapeseed oil and heat over medium-high heat. When the oil is hot, add the tuna and sear for about 2 minutes on each side. You should have a nice crust on the outside and pink raw meat on the inside. Be careful when handling the tuna and try to avoid sticking or tearing the flesh.

6. Place the tuna on a cutting board and with a sharp knife cut it into ¼-inch slices.

7. Combine the broccoli, the ricotta, and about 2 tablespoons of the dressing in a medium bowl. Toss together.

8. Plate the tuna alongside the broccoli, drizzle some additional dressing over the tuna and serve. You can keep the rest of the dressing in the fridge for up to 2 days.

Pan-Seared Salmon with Roasted Brussels Sprouts and Sherry Dressing

This is one of our favorite dinners and has led to a new tradition in our house of "Fish Fridays." After a long week, I always look forward to kicking off the weekend with this decadent yet healthy meal.

DRESSING

1 small shallot, minced

2 tablespoons agave nectar

3 tablespoons sherry vinegar

2 tablespoons balsamic vinegar

3 tablespoons extra-virgin olive oil

¼ cup grapeseed oil

Salt and freshly ground pepper to taste

INGREDIENTS

2 cups trimmed Brussels sprouts

Salt and freshly ground pepper to taste

¼ cup shaved Parmesan cheese

2 salmon fillets (about 5 ounces each)

3 tablespoons grapeseed oil

INSTRUCTIONS

1. Make the dressing: Blend the shallot, agave nectar, sherry vinegar, balsamic vinegar, olive oil, grapeseed oil, salt, and pepper together in a blender.

2. Preheat the oven to 350°F. Bring a large pot of salted water to a boil over high heat.

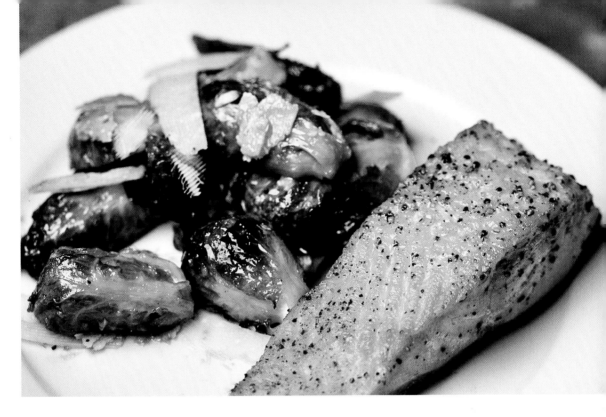

3. Cut the Brussels sprouts lengthwise in half and blanch in the boiling water until slightly softened, about 2 minutes. Drain the Brussels sprouts in a colander and transfer to a large bowl. Add ¼ cup of the dressing and toss to coat. The warm Brussels sprouts will absorb the dressing and soak up the flavors.

4. Spread out the Brussels sprouts in a single layer on a large baking sheet and season generously with salt and pepper. Roast for 25 minutes, shaking the pan occasionally, until they are evenly browned. Remove the Brussels sprouts from the baking sheet and let them cool down in a large bowl while you prepare the fillets. Coat the cooled Brussels sprouts with additional dressing to taste—don't overdo it—and toss with the Parmesan cheese.

5. Coat a large skillet with the grapeseed oil and heat over medium-high heat until it sizzles when you flick water on it. Season the salmon generously with salt and pepper on both sides and place the fillets in the skillet skin side down. Cook for about 4 minutes on each side or until cooked through. Serve with Brussels sprouts.

Salmon Salad–Stuffed Avocado

I love avocado. It's one of my favorite superfoods, not only because it's incredibly good for you but also because of how versatile it is. I love to make avocado the star of my dishes and eat it at breakfast, lunch, and dinner. This refreshing dish pairs smooth, creamy avocado with flavorful salmon salad for a revitalizing dinner or lunch.

INGREDIENTS

2 pan-seared salmon steaks

   (See directions for pan-seared salmon in Pan-Seared Salmon with
   Roasted Brussels Sprouts and Sherry Dressing, page 98.)

½ teaspoon finely chopped fresh dill

6 teaspoons champagne vinegar

Freshly squeezed juice of ½ lemon

4 scallions, finely chopped

Salt and freshly ground pepper to taste

1 large avocado

Cucumber for garnish

Grapefruit for garnish

INSTRUCTIONS

1. In a medium bowl mash the salmon with the dill, vinegar, lemon juice, and scallions until combined.

2. Halve the avocado lengthwise and remove the pit.

3. Split the salmon salad into two equal portions and fill the avocado halves. The salad should stay on top of the avocado. You can garnish with cucumber and a piece of grapefruit.

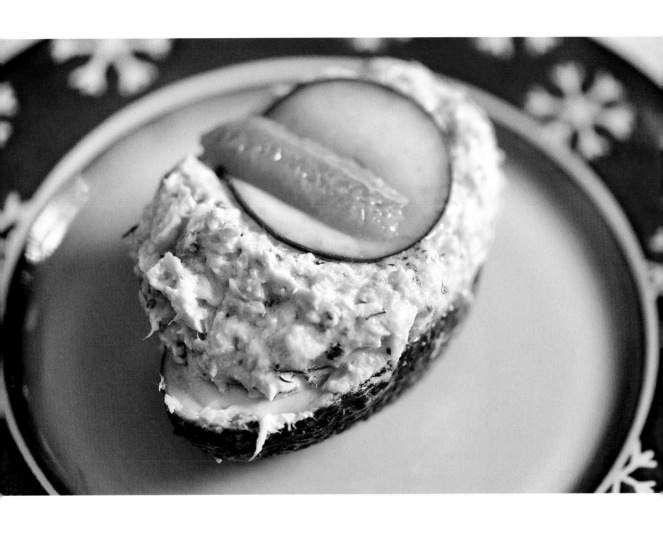

Roasted Sweet Potato with Ground Turkey

This is one of my favorite comfort-yet-healthy foods, and it's absolutely perfect for Thanksgiving dinner. This recipe is WEM, but you can make it FM if you substitute carrots for the sweet potatoes—just cut the roasting time to 13 to 15 minutes.

DRESSING

¼ cup shelled whole pistachios

⅔ cup grapeseed oil

2 tablespoons sherry vinegar

1 tablespoon freshly squeezed orange juice

1 teaspoon freshly squeezed lemon juice

1 teaspoon champagne vinegar

1 small shallot

¼ teaspoon salt

¼ teaspoon freshly ground pepper

INGREDIENTS

1 pound sweet potatoes, unpeeled, scrubbed, and diced into 1-inch cubes

¼ cup extra-virgin olive oil

Salt and freshly ground pepper to taste

1 tablespoon grapeseed oil

1 pound ground turkey

⅓ cup shelled crushed pistachios

½ cup chopped fresh parsley

INSTRUCTIONS

1. Make the dressing: Place the pistachios, grapeseed oil, sherry vinegar, orange juice, lemon juice, champagne vinegar, shallot, salt, and pepper in a blender. Blend on high until smooth.

2. Preheat the oven to 400°F.

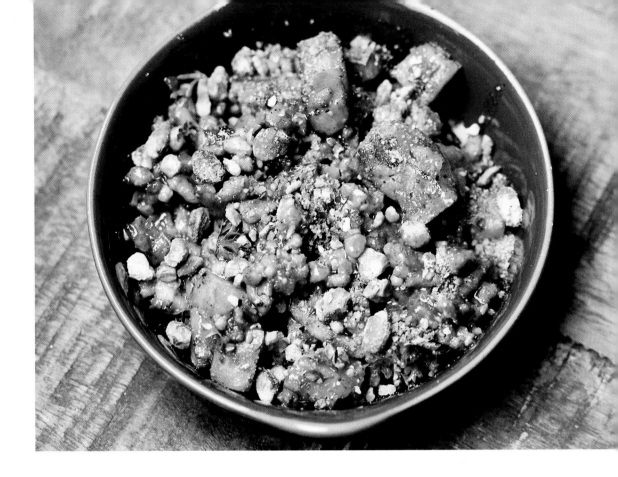

3. Place the sweet potatoes on a large baking sheet, drizzle with the olive oil, and toss to coat. Spread the potatoes into a single layer and season with salt and pepper. Roast for 30 to 40 minutes, turning them every 10 minutes, until they are brown on the outside and tender inside.

4. When the potatoes are almost done, you can start preparing the turkey. Heat the grapeseed oil in a large skillet over medium-high heat and add the turkey. (The oil should sizzle when you add the turkey.) Season with salt and pepper and stir frequently until the turkey is cooked through, about 10 minutes.

5. In a large bowl combine the roasted sweet potatoes, cooked turkey, crushed pistachios, parsley, and about ¼ cup of the dressing. Season with salt and pepper to taste. You can keep the rest of the dressing covered in the fridge. It should stay fresh for about a week.

Sautéed Chicken with Arugula, Strawberries, Blue Cheese, and Sherry Dressing

 This salad is fresh, light, and delicious. The strawberries give this salad the perfect sweetness, but you can swap them for pretty much any fruit that's in season. Grapes are amazing as well!

DRESSING

¼ small shallot

2 tablespoons agave nectar

3 tablespoons sherry vinegar

2 tablespoons balsamic vinegar

3 tablespoons extra-virgin olive oil

¼ cup grapeseed oil

Salt and freshly ground pepper to taste

INGREDIENTS

2 tablespoons grapeseed oil

1 pound skinless boneless chicken breasts, cut into ½-inch strips

Salt and freshly ground pepper to taste

Paprika to taste

1½ cups baby arugula leaves

2 cups sliced fresh strawberries

⅓ cup crumbled blue cheese

INSTRUCTIONS

1. Make the dressing: Place the shallot, agave nectar, sherry vinegar, balsamic vinegar, olive oil, and grapeseed oil in a blender. Blend on high until smooth. Season with salt and pepper.

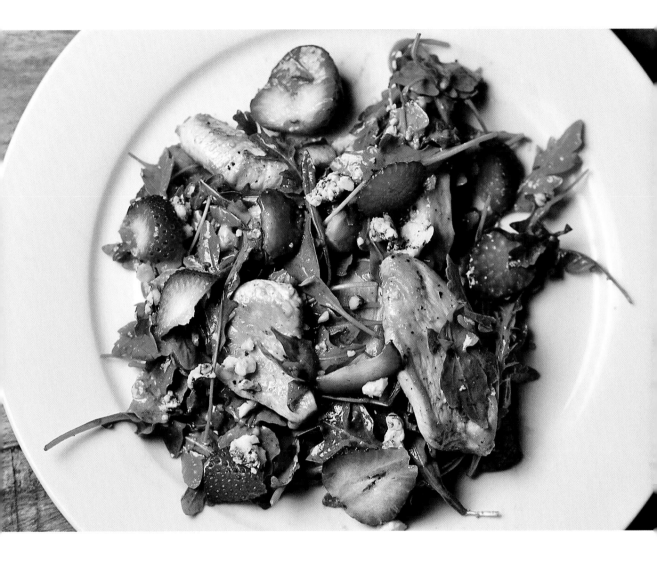

2. Coat a large skillet with a thin layer of the grapeseed oil and heat over medium-high heat. Season the chicken lightly with salt, pepper, and paprika. Sauté, stirring occasionally, until lightly browned all over and cooked all the way through.

3. In a large bowl, mix the arugula with the strawberries, blue cheese, chicken, and about ¼ cup of the dressing.

Ahi Tuna with Cucumber, Mint, Shallots, and Ginger Dressing

This tuna salad makes for a wonderfully light meal that packs a ton of flavor. If you don't want to sauté the steaks, feel free to marinate them for about 30 minutes in freshly squeezed lemon juice to make delicious ceviche.

DRESSING

1 teaspoon grated fresh ginger

1 tablespoon low-sodium soy sauce

1½ teaspoons red wine vinegar

½ teaspoon sesame oil

1 teaspoon agave nectar

1 small garlic clove, minced

½ teaspoon Dijon mustard

½ teaspoon sesame seeds, toasted

½ cup grapeseed oil

Dash of freshly ground pepper, or to taste

INGREDIENTS

3 tablespoons grapeseed oil

Two 6-ounce ahi tuna steaks

Salt and freshly ground pepper to taste

1 large cucumber, chopped into small chunks

4 medium shallots, chopped

¼ cup chopped fresh mint

2 teaspoons white sesame seeds, toasted

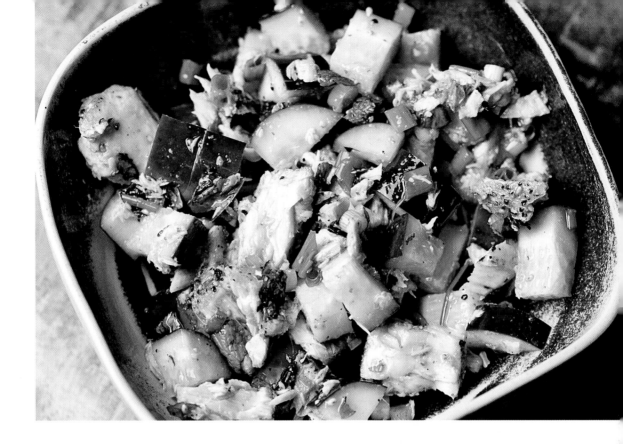

INSTRUCTIONS

1. Make the dressing: Place the ginger, soy sauce, vinegar, sesame oil, agave nectar, garlic, mustard, sesame seeds, grapeseed oil, and pepper in a blender. Blend on high until smooth.

2. Heat the grapeseed oil in a large skillet over medium-high heat. Generously season the tuna with salt and pepper on all sides and place them in the hot oil. (The oil should sizzle when you add the tuna.) Cook the steaks until cooked through, about 4 minutes on a side.

3. Cut the tuna into 1-inch chunks and place them in a large bowl with the cucumber, shallots, mint, sesame seeds, and about 2 tablespoons of the dressing. Mix to combine. Save the rest of the dressing, covered, in the fridge for up to 1 week.

Ceviche

For this recipe it's important that the tuna be fresh. It's worth paying top dollar for the best-quality fish, especially if you're going to eat it basically raw. You can enjoy this Spanish seafood dish for lunch or dinner and know you're eating healthfully!

INGREDIENTS

1 pound ahi tuna

Freshly squeezed juice of 3 lemons

1 medium cucumber, finely diced

2 tablespoons finely chopped fresh mint

¼ cup finely chopped fresh cilantro

1 medium avocado, diced

¼ cup pine nuts

6 scallions, coarsely chopped

DRESSING

2 tablespoons champagne vinegar

1 tablespoon sherry vinegar

2 tablespoons agave nectar

1 tablespoon toasted sesame seeds

Salt and freshly ground pepper to taste

¼ teaspoon chili powder

1 tablespoon olive oil

3 tablespoons grapeseed oil

INSTRUCTIONS

1. Chop the tuna steak into bite-size pieces, place them in a deep glass bowl or dish, and mix with the lemon juice. Cover the dish and place in the refrigerator for 30 minutes.

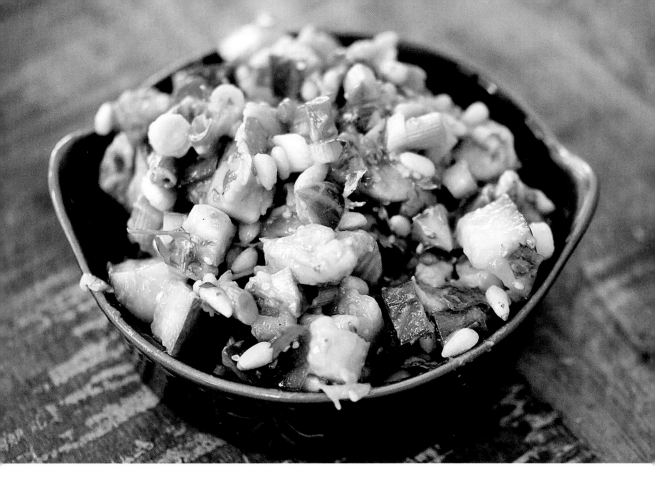

2. Meanwhile, make the dressing: Place the vinegars, agave nectar, sesame seeds, salt and pepper, chili powder, olive oil, and grapeseed oil in a blender and blend on high until smooth.

3. Take the tuna out of the fridge. Drain and discard the lemon juice. Transfer the fish into a medium bowl and combine with the cucumber, mint, cilantro, avocado, pine nuts, and scallions.

4. Toss with about 4 tablespoons of the dressing and store the leftover dressing in the refrigerator. The dressing will last for 3 days in an airtight container. Use it on any salad.

French Toast with a Sunny-Side-Up Egg

This mouth-watering breakfast has it all—sweet, savory yumminess. But it's pretty high in carbs, so make sure you earn it!

INGREDIENTS

3 large eggs

¼ teaspoon ground cinnamon

½ teaspoon agave nectar

1 tablespoon coconut milk

Dash of salt

2 slices of whole-grain bread

1 tablespoon grapeseed oil

2 tablespoons coconut oil

INSTRUCTIONS

1. Crack 2 of the eggs in a deep plate, making sure there's no eggshell floating in the egg whites. Add the cinnamon, agave nectar, coconut milk, and salt; whisk to combine.

2. Add the bread and let it soak in the egg mixture while you heat the grapeseed oil in a medium skillet over medium-high heat.

3. Crack the remaining egg in a small cup, making sure there's no eggshell floating in the egg white. Pour the egg carefully into the hot skillet and try to keep the yolk in the middle of the egg white. Use a spatula to keep the yolk in place. (The oil should sizzle when you add the egg.) Cover and let cook for 1 minute and 50 seconds. Remove from the heat and place the egg carefully on a plate. I like to brown the bottom and edges of my sunny-side-up egg because it adds a light crunch.

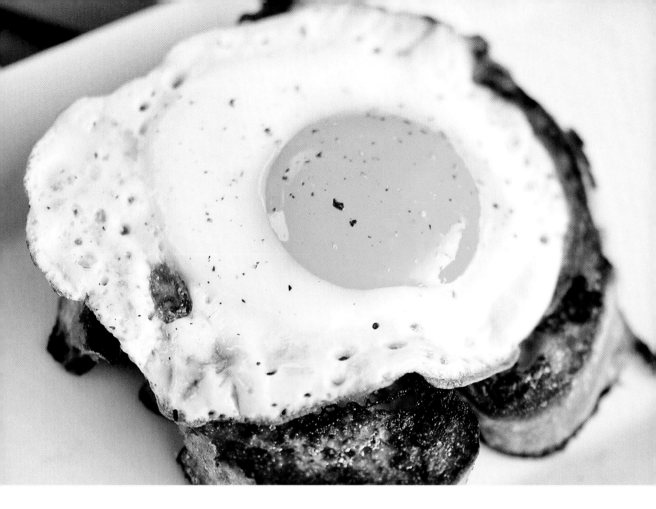

4. Add the coconut oil to the same skillet and heat over medium-high heat. Add the soaked bread to the skillet and cook until both sides are nicely browned, about 1 minute 30 seconds each.

5. Transfer the French toast to the plate with the egg.

Pancakes with Blueberries

This sweet, rich meal is intoxicating to smell as it cooks—you won't be able to stop yourself from sneaking bites. And it's a free meal! This recipe yields four to five good-size pancakes; they're pretty filling and dense in calories, so I usually have just one and share the others around or keep them for a snack.

INGREDIENTS

2 ounces cream cheese

2 large eggs

2 tablespoons erythritol

1 scoop vanilla whey protein powder

⅔ cup almond flour

Pinch of salt

3 tablespoons coconut oil

BLUEBERRY SAUCE

1 teaspoon coconut oil

¼ cup frozen blueberries, thawed

Erythritol to taste (optional)

2 tablespoons whipped cream

INSTRUCTIONS

1. Place the cream cheese, eggs, erythritol, protein powder, almond flour, and salt in the bowl of food processor fitted with the steel blade. Process until you get a smooth batter.

2. In a medium skillet, heat 1 tablespoon of the coconut oil over medium-high heat. Pour ¼ cup batter in the middle of the hot skillet. (The oil should sizzle when you add

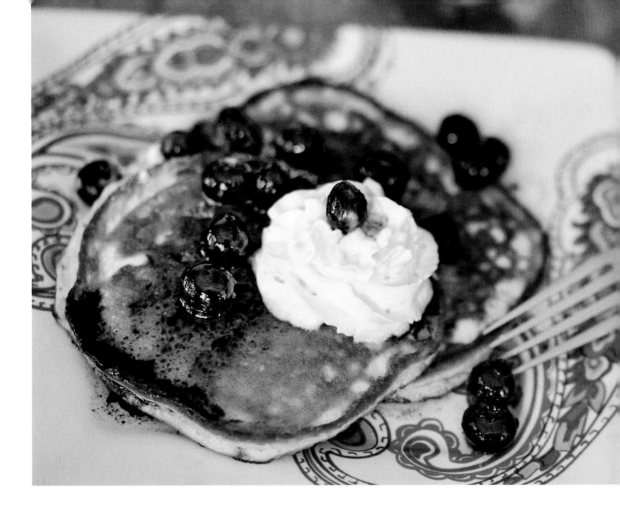

the batter.) Move the skillet gently around until the batter spreads into about a 3-inch circle.

3. Cover and cook until brown, about 1 minute 30 seconds. Uncover and flip the pancake. Cover and cook until brown, 30 to 40 seconds. Repeat until you use all of the batter, adding the remaining coconut oil as needed.

4. When the pancakes are done, make the blueberry sauce: Add the blueberries and coconut oil to the hot skillet. You can sprinkle erythritol over the top, if desired, and cook over medium-high heat, stirring frequently until the blueberries are warm, 3 to 4 minutes.

5. Pour the blueberry sauce over the pancakes and top with the whipped cream.

Breakfast Frittata

This is Jesse's favorite breakfast. It's very light but rich in flavor, and I love that it's so fast and easy to make. It's the perfect breakfast for the entire family. And guess what? Nobody has to earn it with a workout!

INGREDIENTS

6 large egg whites

2 whole large eggs

Salt and freshly ground pepper to taste

½ tablespoon grapeseed oil

2 cups fresh spinach leaves

¼ cup chopped mushrooms

¼ cup chopped broccoli

¼ cup frozen peas and carrots
(mixed frozen veggies; do not thaw)

¼ cup coarsely chopped scallions

½ cup crumbled feta cheese

½ cup ground turkey meat, cooked

INSTRUCTIONS

1. Preheat the broiler.

2. Whisk the egg whites and whole eggs in a medium bowl and season with salt and pepper.

3. Preheat a large cast-iron or ovenproof skillet over medium heat and coat with the grapeseed oil.

4. Add the spinach and sauté for 30 seconds, stirring frequently. Then add the mushrooms, broccoli, peas and carrots, and scallions. Sauté for 1 minute.

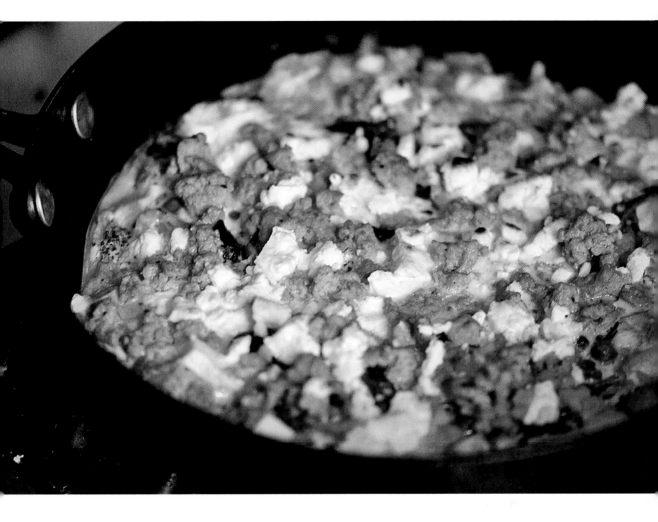

Pour the eggs evenly over the veggies. Cook until the top begins to bubble, 1 to 2 minutes.

5. Spread the feta cheese and turkey evenly over the top. Place the skillet under the broiler for 5 to 10 minutes or until the egg is cooked. It's fine to let the toppings brown a little.

6. Remove from the oven and cut the frittata into 6 wedges; serve warm.

Thai Scramble

If you're bored with regular scrambled eggs, it's time to shake things up with a little bit of Thai flavor. Scrambled eggs have a lot of protein and healthy fat and are very nutritious. Adding ginger and little bit of chili will boost your metabolism and help with digestion. You can never go wrong with this meal, so you don't have to limit yourself to just a breakfast scramble. A midday or evening scramble is just as awesome.

INGREDIENTS

½ tablespoon grapeseed oil

1 teaspoon minced fresh ginger

1 small garlic clove, minced

1 tablespoon sliced scallions

3 large eggs, whisked together in a small bowl

Salt and freshly ground pepper to taste

¼ teaspoon chili powder

1 tablespoon chopped fresh cilantro

INSTRUCTIONS

1. Coat a medium skillet with the grapeseed oil and heat over medium-high heat. Add the ginger, garlic, and scallions. Sauté for 30 seconds and then add the eggs.

2. Cook the eggs, stirring frequently with a spatula and removing the skillet from the heat as necessary to prevent sticking, until the eggs are cooked through. Season with salt, pepper, chili powder, and cilantro.

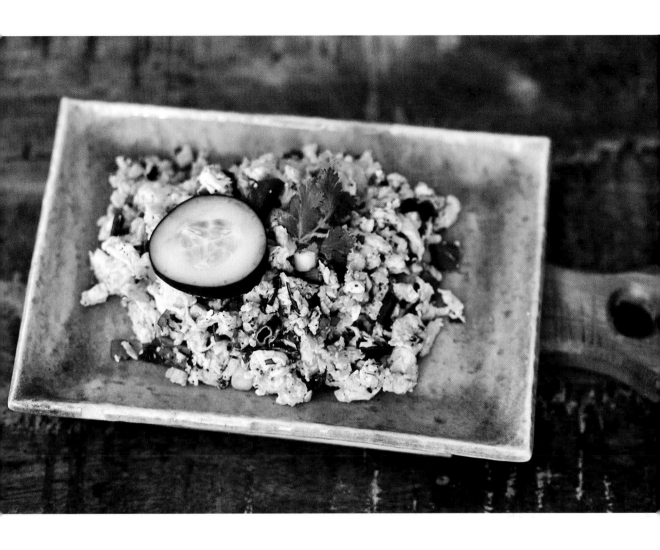

Pecan Apple Oatmeal

Full disclosure: I eat this for breakfast almost every day. That is, every day that I do a workout first thing in the morning, because this way-too-delicious meal is definitely a workout-earned meal. So go ahead, rock your intense workout and earn your scrumptious breakfast. If you go a little bit over the limit with the portion size, it's not a big deal.

INGREDIENTS

1 cup unsweetened almond milk

½ cup rolled old-fashioned oats

½ teaspoon ground cinnamon

½ medium Granny Smith apple, diced

¼ cup crushed pecans

1 tablespoon agave nectar

1 scoop vanilla whey protein powder

INSTRUCTIONS

1. Add ¾ cup of the almond milk to a small saucepan and bring to a boil over medium heat. Add the oats and cinnamon and stir to mix. Reduce the heat to medium-low and simmer, stirring occasionally, 7 to 10 minutes, until the almond milk is absorbed and the oats are soft.

2. Remove from the heat and mix in the apples, pecans, and agave nectar.

3. Combine the remaining ¼ cup of almond milk with the whey protein powder in a blender. Blend on high until smooth.

4. Pour the protein mixture over the oatmeal and serve.

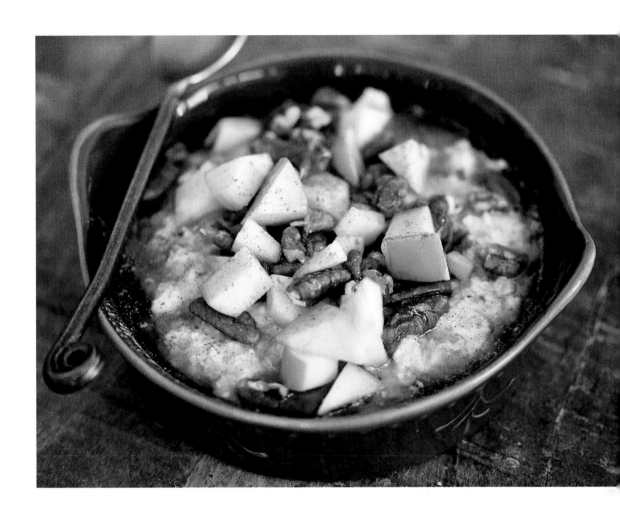

Biscuits

These breakfast biscuits are really simple and fast to make. If you have a sweet tooth and cravings for store-bought, sugar-loaded junk food, you will find this recipe very helpful. I like to munch on three or four of these babies spread with a little bit of grass-fed butter for breakfast, and then I have leftovers for snacks later. If you want, you can add semisweet or dark chocolate chips to the batter and enjoy your homemade chocolate chip biscuits as a post-workout snack.

INGREDIENTS

2½ cups almond flour

½ teaspoon baking soda

2 tablespoons erythritol

15 drops vanilla-flavored stevia

½ teaspoon sea salt

2 large eggs

¼ cup grapeseed oil

1 teaspoon freshly squeezed lemon juice

INSTRUCTIONS

1. Preheat the oven to 350°F. Line a large baking sheet with parchment paper.

2. Combine the almond flour, baking soda, erythritol, stevia, and salt in a large bowl. In a medium bowl, whisk the eggs, grapeseed oil, and lemon juice.

3. Add the egg mixture to the dry ingredients. Work the batter with your hands until thoroughly combined.

4. Place ¼-cup scoops of batter on the prepared baking sheet, placing them 2 inches apart. Don't worry too much about the shape or smoothness of your biscuits—they needn't be perfect.

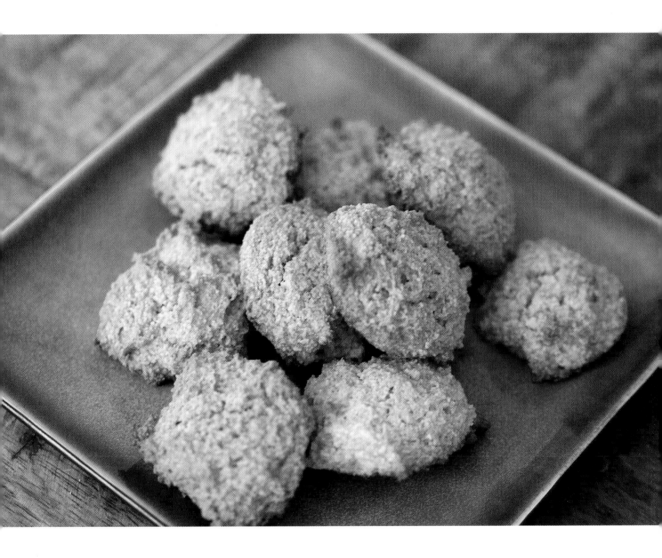

5. Bake for 15 to 25 minutes or until golden brown. Insert a toothpick in the middle of a biscuit; if it comes out clean, remove them from the oven. Store the leftover biscuits in an airtight container in the refrigerator. They should last for 5 days.

Pecan Bread

When you're living the low-carb life, sometimes you just want a good old piece of bread. And I've got some good news for you: While any bread made out of grains is a post-workout meal, breads made from nuts don't have to be earned! You can enjoy them at any time of the day; just add your favorite toppings. I like to keep it simple, and add butter or cheese on top of my nut bread, but you can go as fancy as arugula with goat cheese and a little bit of agave nectar. You can also make a great caprese sandwich. The options are endless. The only thing you have to pay attention to is your portion size, as this bread is quite calorie dense and very filling. I stick to one 1¾-inch-thick slice. The good news is that you can slice the bread and keep it in the freezer in an airtight container; that way you can toast a slice any time of the day. It's always fresh, warm, and crunchy.

INGREDIENTS

Grapeseed oil, for greasing the loaf pan

¼ cup almond flour, plus more for coating the loaf pan

¾ cup roasted almond butter, at room temperature

4 large eggs

¼ teaspoons xanthan gum (a thickener used instead of flour or starch)

1 scoop vanilla whey protein powder

½ teaspoon baking soda

1 teaspoon ground cinnamon

½ teaspoon sea salt

½ cup coarsely chopped pecans

INSTRUCTIONS

1. Preheat the oven to 350°F. Grease a 7 by 3-inch loaf pan with grapeseed oil and flour with almond flour, or use a nonstick loaf pan.

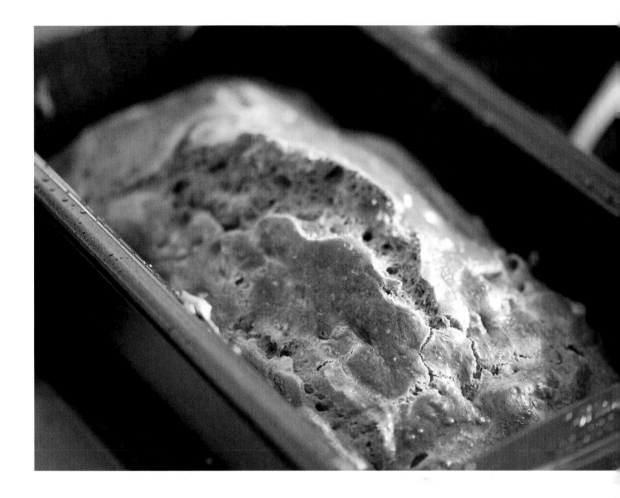

2. In a large bowl, mix the almond butter with the eggs until smooth.

3. In a medium bowl, mix the ¼ cup almond flour, the xanthan gum, protein powder, baking soda, cinnamon, and salt. Add the flour mixture to the almond butter mixture and mix until thoroughly combined. Fold in the pecans and then pour the batter into the prepared pan.

4. Bake for 45 to 50 minutes on the bottom rack of the oven or until a long bamboo stick inserted in the middle of the loaf comes out clean. Let the bread cool in the pan for 1 hour before serving.

Muesli Bread

This bread has a little bit of sweetness to it, but it's still a free meal. Just like the Pecan Bread, it can be sliced and kept in the freezer and you can have a fresh, warm, and crunchy slice any time of the day with your favorite low-carb topping.

INGREDIENTS

Grapeseed oil, for greasing the loaf pan

¾ cup roasted almond butter, at room temperature

1 tablespoon agave nectar

4 large eggs

¼ cup almond flour

¼ teaspoon xanthan gum

½ teaspoon baking soda

1 teaspoon sea salt

1 teaspoon flaxseed meal

¼ cup sesame seeds

¼ cup pepitas

¼ cup walnuts, chopped

¼ cup roasted pistachios

¼ cup dried cranberries

INSTRUCTIONS

1. Preheat the oven to 350°F. Grease a 7 by 3-inch loaf pan. No need to flour the pan.

2. Mix the almond butter, agave nectar, and eggs in a large bowl until smooth.

3. Combine the almond flour, xanthan gum, baking soda, salt, and flaxseed meal in a medium bowl.

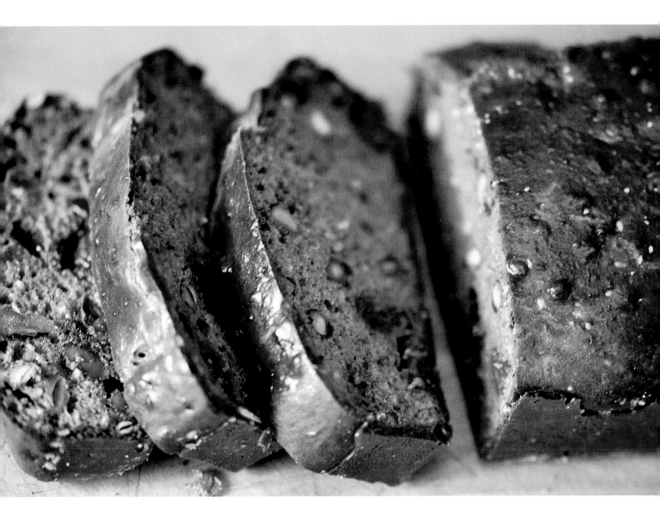

4. Blend the almond flour mixture into the egg mixture until thoroughly combined and then fold in the sesame seeds, pepitas, walnuts, pistachios, and cranberries.

5. Pour the batter into the prepared pan and bake for 50 to 60 minutes, on the bottom rack of the oven, until a long bamboo stick inserted in the middle of the loaf comes out clean. Let the bread cool in the pan for 1 hour before serving. It has to cool before it's removed; otherwise it can break apart.

Roasted Carrots with Sunny-Side-Up Eggs and Bacon

This breakfast is full of flavor and healthy proteins and fats. This recipe yields one portion size, so if you're cooking for a crowd—and trust me, they'll love it—then scale up! It will keep you full for hours and is a great way to start your busy day. The combination of the sunny-side-up egg, carrots, and bacon is simply delicious!

INGREDIENTS

1 cup chopped carrots

1 tablespoon grapeseed oil

Salt and freshly ground pepper to taste

Chili powder to taste

1 strip of bacon

1 large egg

INSTRUCTIONS

1. Preheat the oven to 475°F.

2. Place the chopped carrots on a baking sheet, drizzle with the oil, and toss to coat. Spread them into a single layer. Roast the carrots for 11 minutes. Turn on the broiler and broil the carrots for 2 to 3 minutes. Remove them from the oven and season with salt, pepper, and chili powder.

3. While the carrots are roasting, place the strip of bacon in a large skillet over medium-high heat. Cook until the bacon turns brown and then flip. I like my bacon chewy, so I watch it closely to keep it from browning too much.

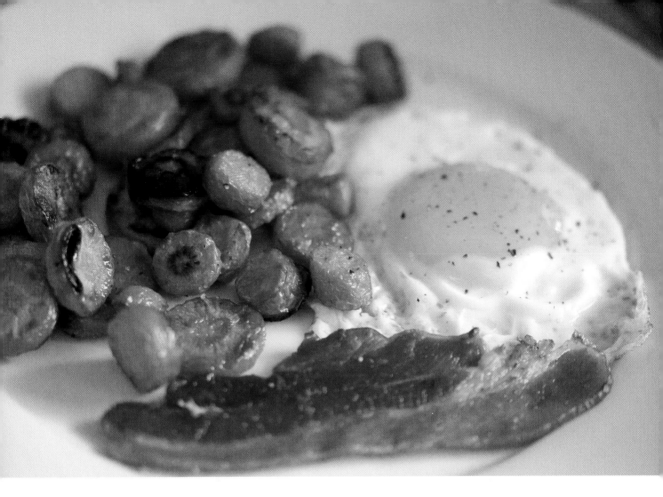

4. Use the bacon fat to cook the egg. Crack the egg into a small cup and make sure that no piece of shell is floating in the egg white. Pour the egg carefully in the hot skillet and try to keep the yolk in the middle of the egg white. (The bacon fat should sizzle when you add the egg.) Cover the pan for about 1 minute. The egg white should be fried at the bottom and solid in the middle, and the egg yolk will be runny when you poke it with a fork—but don't poke it until you're ready to eat it. I like to brown the bottom and edges on my sunny-side-up egg because it adds a light crunch. Remove from the heat and place the egg carefully on a plate. Season the egg with salt and pepper as desired. Serve with the roasted carrots.

Quinoa Bowl with Ground Turkey

This savory and hearty breakfast will stick to your ribs and keep you full all morning. And the best part? You can set the quinoa on to cook and then squeeze in your 15-minute workout while it simmers. Earn and enjoy!

DRESSING

2 tablespoons extra-virgin olive oil

2 teaspoons champagne vinegar

2 teaspoons agave nectar

Pinch of ground cumin

2 tablespoons freshly squeezed lemon juice

Salt and freshly ground pepper to taste

INGREDIENTS

½ cup ground turkey

Salt and freshly ground pepper to taste

¼ cup cooked quinoa

1 chopped medium Granny Smith apple

2 tablespoons chopped red onion

¼ medium avocado

2 tablespoons chopped fresh cilantro

INSTRUCTIONS

1. Make the dressing: Place the olive oil, vinegar, agave nectar, cumin, and lemon juice in a blender. Blend on high until smooth. Season with salt and pepper.

2. Sauté the turkey (no oil needed) in a medium skillet over medium-high heat, stirring to break up any chunks, until cooked through, 6 to 8 minutes. Season with salt and pepper.

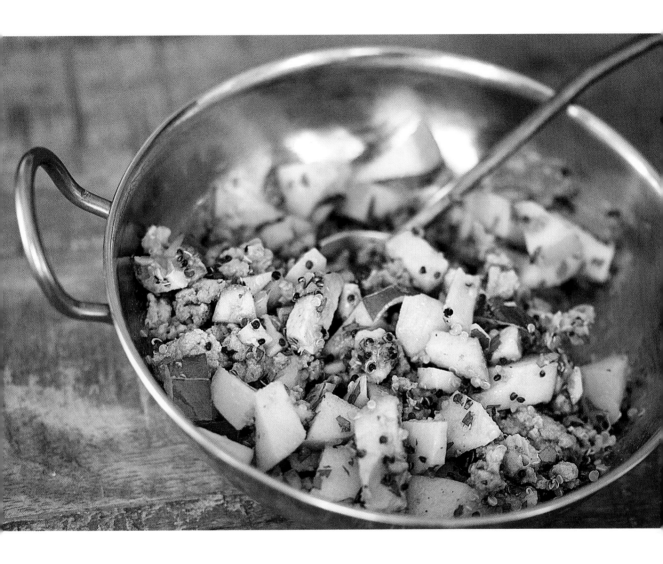

3. Mix the turkey with the quinoa, apple, onion, avocado, and cilantro in a large bowl with 2 tablespoons of the dressing. You can keep the rest of the dressing in the fridge for two days.

Cucumber-Mint Juice

This juice is not only refreshing but can also serve as a low-calorie snack to satisfy your cravings. You'll really love this one in the summer! (Note: this recipe will make a lot!)

INGREDIENTS

2½ cups chopped cucumber

1½ cups coarsely chopped fresh mint

2 cups freshly squeezed lemon juice

1 cup erythritol

3 cups water

Ice for serving

INSTRUCTIONS

1. Place the cucumber, mint, lemon juice, and erythritol in a blender. Blend on high until smooth.

2. Strain the juice through a cloth strainer into a large bowl and then mix in the water.

3. Serve over ice.

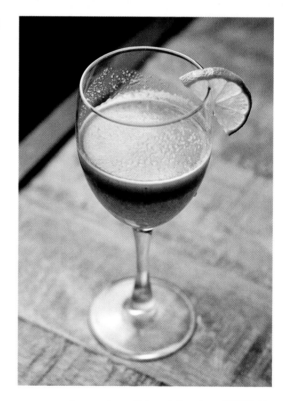

Blueberry-Mint Juice

Fresh, sweet, and actually quite filling. You can use this juice to satisfy your cravings without taking in too many calories.

INGREDIENTS

2 cups frozen blueberries

¾ cup coarsely chopped fresh mint

1 cup erythritol

1 cup freshly squeezed lemon juice

2½ cups water

Ice for serving

INSTRUCTIONS

1. Place the blueberries, mint, erythritol, and lemon juice in a blender. Blend on high until smooth.

2. Strain the juice through a cloth strainer into a large bowl and then mix in the water.

3. Serve over ice.

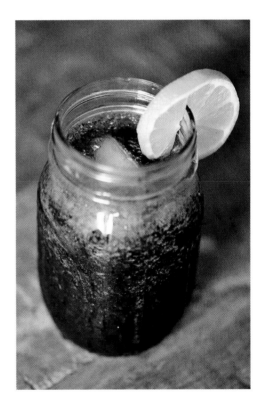

Peach-Ginger Juice

This delicious combo of sweet peaches and spicy ginger makes for a bracing beverage that's refreshing and great for digestion. If your goal is to lose weight, this drink will help you get through the day in between the main meals.

INGREDIENTS

2 cups sliced frozen peaches

1 teaspoon freshly grated ginger

Freshly squeezed juice of ½ lemon

3 tablespoons erythritol

2 cups water

Ice for serving

INSTRUCTIONS

1. Place the peaches, ginger, lemon juice, and erythritol in a blender. Blend on high until smooth.

2. Strain the juice through a cloth strainer into a large bowl and then mix in the water.

3. Serve over ice.

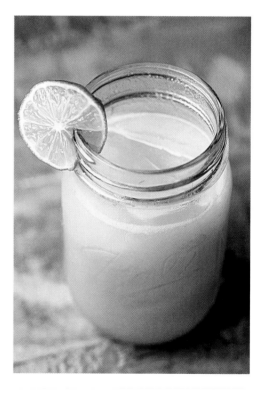

Popeye Smoothie

Spinach made Popeye strong, and it'll do the same for you. This is the ultimate protein shake and a great meal replacement. On a busy day, you can always count on this delicious shake to give you energy and curb your cravings for hours!

INGREDIENTS

1 cup frozen blueberries

1 cup spinach

2 tablespoons sour cream

1 cup unsweetened almond milk

¼ cup whole cashews

1 scoop vanilla whey protein powder

INSTRUCTIONS

1. Place the blueberries, spinach, sour cream, almond milk, cashews, and protein powder in a blender. Blend on high until smooth.

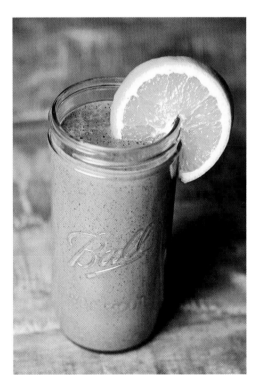

Banana-Peach Frozen Dessert

wem

If you like ice cream, you're going to love this dessert. It's worth earning it with a workout, but if you are really craving it and haven't earned it with a workout, you can always substitute berries for the banana and enjoy this homemade "ice cream" while watching your favorite TV show.

INGREDIENTS

1 frozen medium banana

½ cup sliced frozen peaches

1 teaspoon flaxseed meal

3 tablespoons coconut milk

¼ cup whole or halved macadamia nuts, plus 2 whole nuts for garnish

½ cup unsweetened almond milk

Dash of cinnamon for garnish

INSTRUCTIONS

1. Place the banana, peaches, flaxseed meal, coconut milk, ¼ cup macadamia nuts, and the almond milk in a blender. Blend on high about 30 seconds or until it resembles a thick frozen dessert.

2. Pour into a bowl and garnish with a dash of cinnamon and a couple of macadamia nuts.

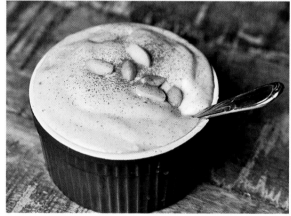

Vanilla Chia Pudding

When you put chia seeds in liquid, they slowly absorb the moisture and flavor of whatever they're in. In this dish, they turn into a delicious, thick, filling vanilla pudding. The only downfall of this snack is that you'll want to have too much of it. Eat slowly and stay lean!

INGREDIENTS

½ scoop vanilla whey protein powder

½ cup unsweetened almond milk

2 tablespoons chia seeds

¼ cup mixed fresh blueberries, raspberries, strawberries (if you have only one kind of berry, that will suffice)

INSTRUCTIONS

1. Mix the protein powder and almond milk in a small bowl. Place the chia seeds in a small glass, add the milk mixture, and stir to combine. Let it chill in the refrigerator for 1 hour. The chia seeds will absorb the almond milk and soften, which creates the delicious pudding.

2. Stir in the berries and serve in a large glass.

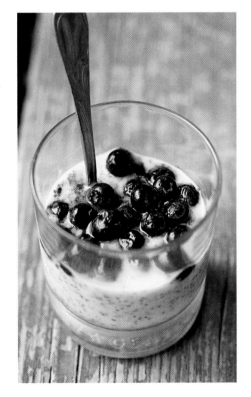

Baked Parmesan Zucchini Sticks

This is a healthy comfort food that you don't have to earn. When you're hankering for fish sticks or French fries, turn to this instead to satisfy your fried food craving.

INGREDIENTS

1 large zucchini

1 large egg

Salt and freshly ground pepper to taste

½ cup almond flour

¼ cup flaxseed meal

½ cup finely shredded Parmesan cheese

Mayonnaise (optional)

INSTRUCTIONS

1. Preheat the oven to 425°F. Line a baking sheet with parchment paper.

2. Slice the zucchini in half and then slice each half in to 3 equal sticks.

3. Crack the egg into a pie plate or other deep plate and whisk. Season with salt and pepper.

4. Combine the almond flour, flaxseed meal, and Parmesan cheese in a deep plate.

5. Dip each zucchini stick in the egg and then coat with the almond flour mixture.

6. Place the zucchini sticks 2 inches apart on the prepared pan and bake for 20 minutes or until they turn golden. Serve plain or with mayo.

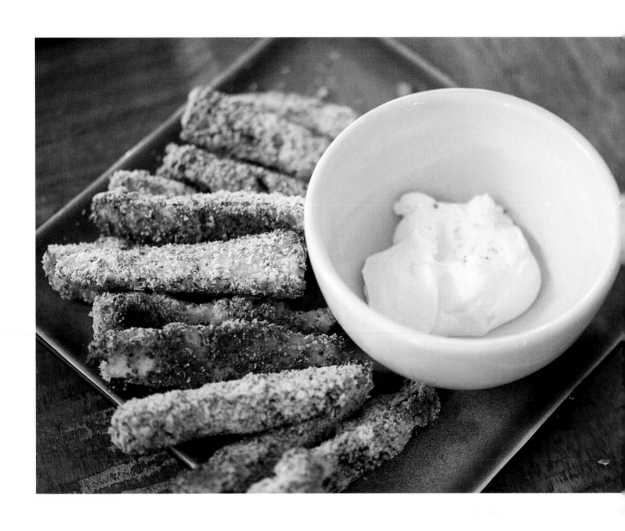

Pecan Toast with Apple, Carrot, and Pecans

There are hundreds of ways you can have your toasted pecan bread. This is just one of them that I really enjoy. Who says that a low-carb diet can't be satisfying and delicious?

INGREDIENTS

1 slice frozen Pecan Bread (page 122)

1 medium Granny Smith apple

1 large carrot

2 tablespoons chopped pecans

1 teaspoon honey

Scant ¼ teaspoon ground cinnamon

INSTRUCTIONS

1. Preheat the oven to 350°F. Toast the Pecan Bread in the oven for 8 minutes or in a toaster. It should be crispy on the top and bottom and hot on the inside.

2. Place the apple and carrot in a blender. Blend on high until shredded but not smooth.

3. Transfer the apple mixture to a small bowl. Add the pecans and honey and mix until combined.

4. Spoon all of the apple-nut mixture on top of the toast and enjoy.

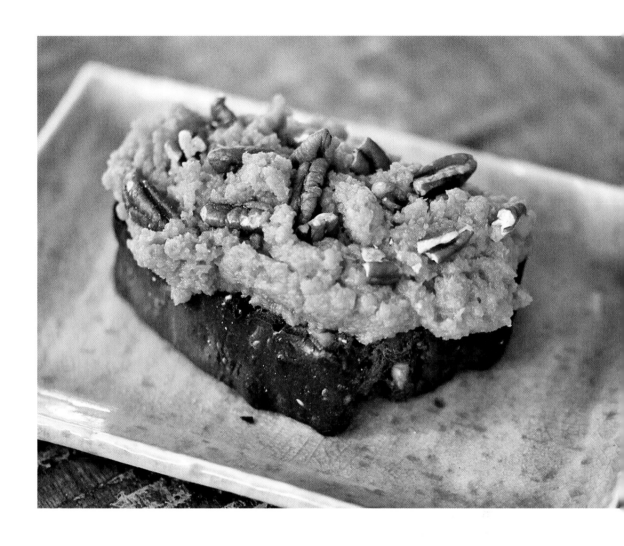

Protein Power Balls

Finally, a delicious dessert that doesn't require any cooking or baking! You can throw this recipe together in minutes, and it will give you sustainable energy for hours. I have one or two balls as a snack in between meals. It's not going to be easy to stick to a small portion size because they taste like heaven, so you'll have to stay strong—or earn it first, then pig out.

INGREDIENTS

⅓ cup whole pistachios

⅓ cup whole walnuts

⅓ cup whole cashews

½ scoop vanilla whey protein powder

1 teaspoon unsweetened cocoa powder

2 tablespoons coconut oil

1 tablespoon agave nectar

2 tablespoons shredded unsweetened coconut

INSTRUCTIONS

1. Place the pistachios, walnuts, cashews, protein powder, and cocoa in a blender. Blend on high until almost smooth; the consistency should be mostly like a nut flour with small pieces of nuts still visible.

2. Transfer the nut mixture to a medium bowl and add the coconut oil and agave nectar; combine thoroughly, using your hands, to make a uniform mixture.

3. Place the coconut into a small bowl.

4. Roll the nut mixture into small even-size balls and dip each one in the shredded coconut. Store the nut balls in an airtight container in the fridge for a week.

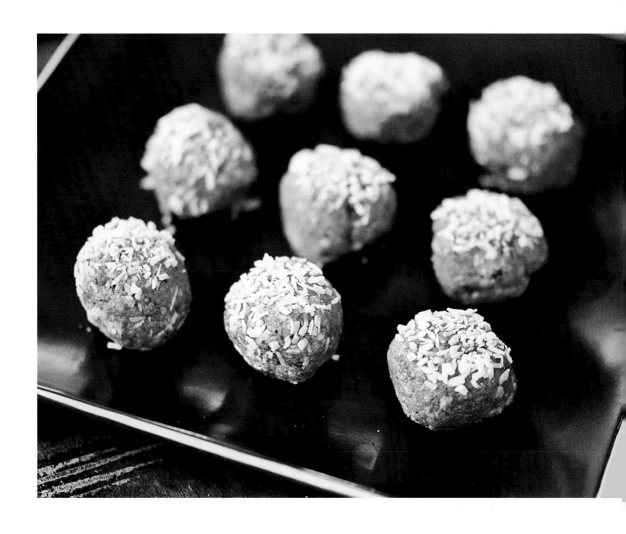

Zuzka's Deviled Eggs

If you're a fan of deviled eggs, wait till you taste these. This is my favorite deviled eggs recipe in the world, and I love that I get to use more exciting ingredients instead of just mayo. It's also a great snack that you don't have to earn with your workout. Enjoy it any time, but watch your portion size. These quantities are perfect for one serving.

PISTACHIO DRESSING

- ¼ cup shelled whole pistachios
- ⅔ cup grapeseed oil
- 2 tablespoons sherry vinegar
- 1 tablespoon freshly squeezed orange juice
- 1 teaspoon freshly squeezed lemon juice
- 1 teaspoon champagne vinegar
- ¼ small shallot
- ¼ teaspoon salt
- ¼ teaspoon freshly ground pepper

INGREDIENTS

- 1 large hard-boiled egg
- ½ tablespoon cream cheese
- Salt and freshly ground pepper to taste
- 2 walnut halves for garnish
- Paprika to taste

INSTRUCTIONS

1. Make the dressing: Place the pistachios, grapeseed oil, sherry vinegar, orange juice, lemon juice, champagne vinegar, shallot, salt, and pepper in a blender. Blend on high until smooth.

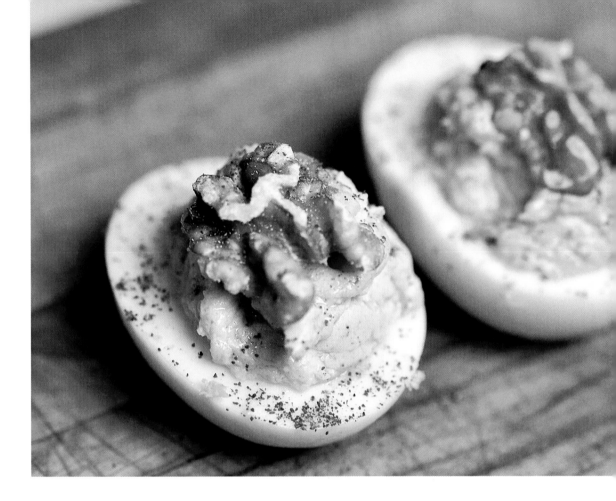

2. Slice the hard-boiled egg in half lengthwise and remove the yolk. Set the whites aside.

3. Thoroughly combine the yolk with 1 tablespoon of the pistachio dressing and cream cheese in a small bowl, mixing with a fork until smooth. Add salt and pepper to taste.

4. Divide the yolk mixture equally between the 2 egg whites and top each with a walnut half. Sprinkle with paprika.

Staying Healthy at Parties

No holiday celebrates healthy eating. Instead, we have Christmas cookies, Thanksgiving feasts, Halloween candy, Fourth of July barbecue, Valentine's Day chocolates, and New Year's champagne toasts. The celebrations in between them are also more about indulgence than clean eating.

When we cheat and splurge on fatty, sugary, not-so-healthy things, returning to a nutritious diet only becomes more difficult. I want you to try to stick to your diet and routine because being fit and healthy is worth celebrating! Here are some tips to help you avoid those party foods, especially during the holidays.

- Eat a light meal at home before leaving for the party. When you arrive, you won't make a beeline for the snack tray. Protein and fiber will keep you full much longer too! Skipping meals will only make you hungrier.
- So far, so good. Now grab a sparkling water! Wait 30 minutes to snack. Relax and survey your food choices. Hit the veggie or fruit trays. No gut bombs there.
- If you don't love it, don't eat it! Skip the items that are available all year long.
- Chew gum or have a mint.
- Alternate alcohol with water, halving your beverage calories in the process.
- If you're bringing food, bring something healthful. At least you'll know there's one nutritious item you can eat at the party.
- Put food on a napkin! At parties, there are usually plates—small or large—but a napkin holds only a limited amount of food. Sneaky—but it works.

My Workout Philosophy:
Short and Sweat

My basic workout methodology consists of short, super-intense workouts done nearly every day—and if you're looking for real transformation, then every day. When the workouts take only 15 minutes to complete, it's easy to find time in your daily schedule to break a good sweat. During that time you will train your entire body, not just part of it, and you will be doing resistance training at the same time as you're doing cardio. What's more, all of the workouts in this book consist of body weight exercises. No equipment needed. However, I'll warn you now: My workouts are effective only with maximum effort. You have to push yourself to complete as many reps as possible in 15 minutes. There won't be time for drinking water or chatting with your friend.

This may differ from the other training approaches you've encountered so far in your fitness life. In fact, every single point I made in the preceding paragraph might contradict information you've heard before, starting with "super-intense workouts."

I haven't set foot in a gym in eight years, but I remember it being a social setting as much as a place of exercise. Some people enjoy that scene; they want to spend an hour or more in the gym every day. It's their chance to see friends, make small talk, and maybe get in a workout. Sure, maybe they're in there for an hour, but all told, they probably don't work out longer than I do. Personally, I would rather focus on my workout for 15 minutes and then spend my spare time somewhere other than the gym.

You're probably also used to hearing this mantra from bodybuilding or fitness magazines: *You must take rest days between workouts. If you train biceps, you must wait 48 hours before you lift so much as a pencil again.* That sort of thing. Well, if you go to the gym and do 16 sets only for biceps, your arms probably *do* need rest. But that's not what we're doing here. We're not trying to develop big, bulky muscles; we're trying to get fit for life. These workouts will involve your whole body, not just one area, so there won't be any particular muscle dying for rest. And if you use your non-workout time for appropriate recovery, as I'll outline in Chapter 10, you'll be fine. With total fitness and full recovery as the goals, training for 15 minutes a day every day is not excessive. Muscle fibers aren't being annihilated as they are during a body-building workout. To support this style of training, you need plenty of sleep and a healthy diet—but you need those things anyway.

I also like frequent training because it hard-wires working out into a fitness habit. If you're training only several times a week, by default you'll have a day or two off. Some might say that allows people to stick with their workouts, but I think the opposite. You're always a missed workout or two away from sliding back into not training at all. In my system, training becomes as routine as brushing your teeth or going to work. To paraphrase Nike, you just do it.

The idea that you will be training your entire body may also seem alien. The mainstream approach to working out has its roots in bodybuilding, which was interpreted for the masses for many years in magazines such as *Muscle & Fitness* and *Muscular Development*. Most of the workouts focused on particular muscles or muscle groups, such as biceps, pectorals, quads, hamstrings, and abs. The workouts were designed to make those muscles grow bigger and in proportion to one another. This made sense for competitive bodybuilders who were judged onstage based on conditioning, symmetry, and proportion. Standing there in their posing trunks, they knew that even a slight deficit in, say, their trapezius or rear deltoids could lower their ranking.

I prefer to emphasize total fitness and well-rounded conditioning. To me, the whole is not just the sum of its parts; the whole is what matters, first and foremost. Games and matches aren't won or lost with one muscle group, and certainly life situations aren't body-part specific. You need muscles, but you also need coordination, endurance, agility, and other qualities. My workouts build those attributes simultaneously.

The idea of doing resistance training at the same time as you're doing cardio may also seem different to you. Again, the traditional approach is to do weights one day and cardio the next. I like to mix them together so my heart rate is elevated while my muscles are working. Not only is this efficient but it also develops strength under duress. The stereotype is of the bodybuilder who has tons of muscle but who can't run around the block without huffing or puffing. I want to be at my strongest when I need strength the most, and that's probably going to be on a playing field or court or in an emergency situation in real life. People who follow my plan will be training for life, and they will be equipped to deploy their skills in emergencies if necessary.

This phrase might also come as a revelation: My workouts are effective only if you give maximum effort. Make no mistake, you will be working very hard during each 15-minute stretch. The lack of rest in particular may shock your system. If you don't put forth enough effort, those 15 minutes can't work their magic. I see this a lot when people are doing high-intensity interval training (HIIT). *HIIT* is defined as short, anaerobic bursts of exercise followed by a brief rest; the sequence is repeated several times. Usually a HIIT session takes 15 to 20 minutes. They don't last any longer than that because high-intensity intervals are very demanding.

Many people underestimate how hard you have to work during the work interval to generate the benefits found in the studies touting HIIT's greatest benefits. They think they're working hard enough, but they're not. You *really* have to push it with HIIT, and you *really* have to push it with my workouts too.

Challenges and AMRAPs

My 15 Minutes to Fit workout plan consists of 15 AMRAPs, which stands for "as many rounds as possible." What that means is, I want you to go as hard as you can—and I realize that, initially, you may not be able to complete the entire workout on a given day. However, while the time stays the same—15 minutes—the volume of work completed increases as you go. It should increase, anyway. The good news, especially for beginners, is the workout duration is fixed. You know it's not going to take 30 minutes; you have only 15; and if the workout lasts only 15 minutes, you want to maximize that window, and so you push yourself that much harder.

Expect a learning curve with my workouts. Not only are you being taxed physically but you may be doing these exercises for the first time. Don't worry if you struggle a bit at first. Let's say a workout calls for three rounds, and at the 15-minute mark, you've completed only two and a half. As long as you keep moving through the whole workout, you'll still reap at least some and perhaps most of the benefits of my workouts, even if you don't complete as many reps as a more experienced person.

The next time you do that same workout, I challenge you to better your previous effort by doing more work in the same amount of time. Seeing the time wind down before your eyes makes it easier to push yourself harder. The workout's going to become more effective and more challenging. And it makes it more fun because you have a very simple goal in mind.

Some people are more competitive than others, needless to say, but everyone can benefit from this approach. I really enjoy it because I feel like I have a purpose when I work out, above and beyond just looking great. Better to take the focus off that aspect and just focus on the performance aspect.

HIIT Training

My workouts may remind you of HIIT, albeit with my own Z twist. HIIT is now proven to be one of the most effective methods to shape up and improve athletic performance. Here are three reasons out of many why HIIT produces such great results:

1. *HIIT is incredibly time-efficient.* The intensity of HIIT requires that workouts be relatively short. No more long, boring workouts that can take one to two hours. These longer, less intense workouts often yield poor results by comparison and are less efficient regarding time and energy output.

2. *HIIT workouts not only increase your aerobic capacity but also increase your anaerobic capacity.* In comparison, jogging increases only your aerobic capacity. A recent study found a 14 percent increase in aerobic capacity from six weeks of HIIT, whereas in the same study, six weeks of jogging provided only a 9 percent increase in aerobic capacity. The same study showed virtually no improvement in anaerobic capacity from jogging, while HIIT provided a 28 percent improvement in anaerobic capacity!

3. *HIIT workouts blast your metabolism and burn more fat and calories compared to steady-state aerobic activities such as running or cycling.* In fact, HIIT continues to burn fat even after the workout ends. According to a study in the *Journal of Applied Physiology*, women experienced a 30 percent increase in fat oxidation after performing seven HIIT workouts over a two-week period. Fat oxidation is a key indicator of fat loss. HIIT also triggers the release of human growth hormone, a substance essential for building muscle.

Your Return on Investment

I'm asking you to invest 15 minutes of every day in yourself by working out. For many of you, the reward will be weight loss and a better-looking body. That's really only the beginning, though. Fitness has benefits that influence your health, your career, and your entire life—really.

Exercise and Health

Exercise and Menopause

Some of you may either be going through menopause or fast approaching it. Most women reach menopause in their 40s and 50s. The average age of onset in the United States, according to the Mayo Clinic, is 51 years old. As the term suggests, menopause signals the natural end of a woman's menstrual cycles. This ending is often accompanied by mood swings, hot flashes, depression, weight gain, low energy, and a variety of other disconcerting physical and emotional symptoms. Their severity and duration vary by individual. I know, I know, sounds like a lot of fun, huh?

While there are no magic answers to remedying the variety of symptoms associated with menopause, women can take steps to lessen the impact of menopause on their lives. According to the authors of the book *Mind over Menopause*, exercise can dramatically curb menopause symptoms. Three key takeaways:

1. A Swedish study found that the number of moderate and severe hot flashes for women in the study who consistently exercised was almost *half* that of women who didn't. Hey, if you're going to sweat anyway, you might as well do it while working out!

2. As for depression and anxiety, exercise also can have a pronounced effect on stabilizing your mood due to all the feel-good chemicals that flood your brain. As well, exercise can allow your mind to better handle stress and find your way out of the menopausal fog.

3. Finally, and most obviously, consistently exercising can limit or even stop the weight gain that many women experience during menopause.

Exercise and Alzheimer's

Recent studies done at Georgia Tech University and the Cleveland Clinic in Ohio demonstrate the beneficial role exercise has on memory and, potentially, curbing the effects of dementia and Alzheimer's in aging individuals.

The study done at Georgia Tech demonstrated that lifting weights improved long-term memory upward of 10 percent in healthy, young adults. This particular study focused on weightlifting. Previous studies had already demonstrated that aerobic exercise such as running and walking improved memory as well. All the more reason to work out before a big exam!

The Cleveland Clinic study focused on the role exercise may play in preventing, or at least limiting, the effects of Alzheimer's disease in elderly individuals. The results were startling and quite encouraging. Alzheimer's disease changes the physical landscape of the brain, causing memory loss and dementia. However, this particular study showed that exercise also changes the physical makeup of the brain, potentially limiting the negative effects of Alzheimer's. Exercise did not cure individuals, but according to the researchers, it may very well limit or lessen the effects of the disease. More research is needed to provide conclusive evidence.

Exercise and Bone Health

According to the Harvard School of Public Health, osteoporosis occurs in 80 percent of all menopausal women! Menopause may be a long way off for some of you, but plan ahead. Building and maintaining healthy bones now will pay off later. Osteoporosis is a preventable disease and not something we have to live in fear of as we age. We can and should take the necessary steps to ensure that our bones remain strong throughout our entire life.

Exercise is crucial for bone health and the prevention of osteoporosis. Weight-bearing exercises, including body weight exercises, puts a beneficial stress on our bones, which triggers growth. This growth forces our bones to become denser and stronger. It's a cliché, but an ounce of prevention is indeed worth a pound of cure.

Exercise and Anxiety

The average hectic weekday is filled with anxiety. Early morning commutes, screaming kids, overbearing bosses, and impossible deadlines surround us. The more we try to tell ourselves to just relax, the more impossible it seems. We take a few deep breaths hoping for a miracle, but our anxieties still stand before us like thugs in some gangster movie.

Anxiety feels debilitating, making us stumble throughout our day. It can also drive us to make poor choices without realizing it. Rather than soothing our anxieties, lifestyle choices like eating junk food, lounging around, and drinking heavily end up making our anxieties even worse.

The right choice when dealing with anxiety and stress is often the tougher, harder choice. For example, you just ended your workday. You're beat. Your boss's condescending demands are still ringing in your ears. Your drive home was even longer than expected due to a congested river of freeway traffic, and apparently using turn signals has gone the way of the dinosaurs. Your mind and body are demanding that you relax, relax, relax. The trouble is, you can't. It seems impossible. You're overflowing with anxious energy.

What scientific research now demonstrates more and more is that consistent physical activity is perhaps the most effective balm you can use to calm your frayed nerves. Of course, it seems almost illogical after a long, exhausting day to blast through a 20-minute HIIT routine or even go for a three-mile run, but in fact it's not.

Elizabeth Gould, PhD, a neuroscientist who runs the Gould Lab at Princeton University, recently published a study indicating that people who consistently exercise develop a much more effective neurological response when dealing with stress and anxiety. Aside from all the feel-good chemicals that are released during exercise, the brains in people who consistently work out may actively soothe them during moments of anxiety. This may lessen the duration of such stress.

Gould's study focused on the brain's hippocampus region, which is largely responsible for our emotions. Her findings indicated that continuous exercise may reshape this area of the brain in a manner that allows people to cope with and manage stress and anxiety in a far better way than those who choose a sedentary lifestyle.

It's hard not to freak out when you're anxious, but try to channel that energy into your workouts. You'll feel the difference over time. Plenty of research supports this, and so do I!

Exercise and Stress

Stress can have a terrible effect on us. It can make us anxious and irritable, frustrated and depressed. Worse, sometimes these moods can linger longer than expected. The mental strain that stress causes can lead to physical symptoms as well. Muscles tense up, causing headaches or back pain; our immune system weakens, leading to illnesses such as constant bouts of colds or flu. Over time, stress can even contribute to life-threatening illnesses such as heart disease and cancer.

The good news is that when we physically stress our bodies with exercise, it actually *relieves* our mental and emotional stress. Working out may be the perfect antidote to stressful times. Not only does exercise help us deal with stress, but there are plenty of clinical studies that now demonstrate how exercise also can help with mood disorders such as anxiety and depression.

According to researchers at Harvard, exercise plays an important role in physiologically limiting our body's natural responses to emotional stress. Consistently working out has been shown to dramatically reduce the levels of hormones triggered by stress. Exercise also biochemically stimulates our body's natural painkillers and mood enhancers in the form of endorphins and norepinephrine. What's more, it stimulates our brain and improves our cognitive abilities.

Over time, consistent exercise also teaches our bodies to be better at stress management. A recent report by the American Psychological Association explained that exercise forces the various systems in our bodies—cardiovascular, nervous, muscular, and so on—to communicate with greater precision with one another. This allows us to physiologically handle stress in a more efficient and productive manner compared to individuals who remain sedentary.

Exercise also provides behavioral changes that help manage stress. When we consistently focus on fitness and well-being and make it an essential part of who we are, our self-image improves. Our muscles develop and grow. Our waistlines shrink as we burn off fat. We fit better in our clothes. More important, we *feel* better. We have more energy. This has a dramatic effect on our psyche, generating a more positive outlook toward ourselves and toward life.

Exercise also provides a nice distraction from our busy, often stressful lives. When we physically push ourselves to exhaustion, we have little choice but to focus on the task at hand. This requirement of focus serves as a positive distraction from our problems and lets us come back to them with at least a little more objectivity than we had before.

Exercise and Depression

Sometimes the blues just won't leave. Dark clouds linger around us and little can brighten our days. No wonder pharmaceutical companies are making a fortune off our sorrows. I went through a major depressive period myself that lasted a year and a half. Exercise was one of the things that kept me sane.

Thankfully, a study out of Duke University offers compelling evidence that at least 30 minutes of brisk, cardiovascular exercise a day is more effective than taking Zoloft, a common drug therapy for depression. The study also demonstrated that the more one exercised, the less likely it was that depression would return. Another startling conclusion was that taking an antidepressant had no added benefits to simply exercising.

Why does exercise work in treating depression? Gary Small, MD, a professor of psychiatry and biobehavioral sciences at the University of California, Los Angeles, suggests that exercise increases blood flow to the brain and releases endorphins, our body's natural antidepressants. If you've ever felt euphoric after a workout, chances are that your body let loose a healthy dose of endorphins.

Exercise releases serotonin as well as endorphins. Aside from factors such as grief and loss, many in the scientific community believe a lack of serotonin is the main culprit in triggering depression. In fact, antidepressant drugs often increase serotonin production in the brain.

A great experiment to do with yourself when you are feeling down or anxious is to work out or go for a light jog for 30 to 60 minutes. Immediately afterward, gauge your mood. More than likely, you'll feel a palpable lift to your spirits and mood. It may require a bit more willpower to get yourself going if you're unhappy or stressed, but it'll be worth it. Exercise, rather than taking a pill, can provide us with a greater sense of control over our daily stresses and sorrows. It can also teach us that our lives do not have to be at the mercy of our moods. Instead, we can actually control how we feel with effort and persistence and take better charge of our lives.

Five Surprising Benefits of Exercise

1. *You will sleep better.* Nothing makes you sleep better than a good workout. Your body is able to use the downtime for the tissue-repair work that keeps you both looking and feeling great.

2. *You will have a faster metabolism.* A recent study done at Appalachian State University showed that 45 minutes of vigorous cycling elevated the participants' basal metabolic rate (BMR) for up to 14 hours. BMR determines how many calories you would burn if you just stayed in bed all day. So if you increase your BMR, you're burning more calories even when you're not working out. This is one of the keys to weight loss!

3. *You will build stronger bones.* As we age, our bones lose much of their density. We can put a brake on that process by working out with weights to build bone mass.

4. *You will age more gracefully.* Consistent exercise helps you maintain a young, vibrant look. Exercise is the largest contributor to growth hormone release, which is known for slowing down the aging process and promoting youth and vitality.

5. *Your skin will be clear and vibrant.* Two recent studies done at McMaster University in Canada demonstrated that exercise not only prolonged healthy skin, it often reversed damage caused by age. So go ahead and sweat it out with me! Exercise is the real fountain of youth!

CHAPTER 9

The 15 Minutes to Fit Workout Plan

My workout routines seem really short. Is 15 minutes a day really enough to get visible results? Absolutely. This is how I've been keeping myself in awesome shape for the past seven years, and research increasingly supports the benefits of short, high-intensity workouts. These workouts are extremely effective for building strength, increasing stamina, and burning tons of calories. Besides that, you will see visible results really soon if you stay consistent and support your training with a healthy diet. I'm in better shape now than I was in my early twenties, thanks to my workouts and my lifestyle.

No Pain, No Gain

I'm sure many of you have experienced the following painful symptoms when working out hard. Your muscles feel like they might be caught in some kind of exercise-induced wildfire from all the lactic burn. Suddenly oxygen seems to be at a premium.

Your lungs are caught in a bear hug and maybe you're even a little nauseated. Your timer or stopwatch could not be moving any slower, and if you have to do one more squat you're pretty sure you might turn into Jell-O and collapse onto the floor.

I'll be the first to tell you that working out effectively and consistently is not easy. In fact, it can be a downright pain in the behind. Some of you may laugh a little if I tell you that consistently working out is actually good for managing the aches and pains in our bodies, but it's true!

Scientists are well aware that strenuous exercise temporarily increases our resistance to pain. As I mentioned, our bodies release natural painkillers in the form of endorphins during tough workouts. A whole host of studies seem to indicate that, at least for a short duration of time, working out greatly increases our tolerance for pain; this phenomenon is known as *exercise-induced hypalgesia*.

Still, what about the long-term effects of exercise on pain management? After all, we are trying to focus on longevity and well-being, not just looking good (though that helps!). A recent study done at the University of New South Wales and Neuroscience Research Australia indicates that one of the more pronounced effects of consistent exercise is a substantial increase in tolerating pain long-term as well.

While the study was unable to find an exact physiological reason for the increase in pain tolerance, it did discover that working out develops mental fortitude and toughness to better handle pain. However, PhD student Matthew Jones, the lead researcher in the study, believes that the brain is providing some kind of neurological response as well. This neurological response seems likely given how much research has come out as of late regarding exercise and the brain.

Of course, if you're injured or feeling a sharp pain anywhere in your body, go see a doctor immediately. Otherwise, get ready to chase those aches and pains away with me!

The 15 Minutes to Fit Workout Plan

For every workout, the goal is to do as many rounds as possible in 15 minutes. Rest only as needed between sets; ideally you won't rest at all, although it may take time for you to reach that conditioning level. Keep cycling through the moves listed for that day. So for Day 1, perform 20 jump squats, followed by 10 push-ups, and so on. Once you've done one set of each of the five exercises, that's one round.

Where you read the symbol "×" followed by a number, I'm asking you to perform that number of repetitions—say, 10, for example. If you read a number followed by "alt." (meaning "in alternating fashion"), I want you to switch back and forth between limbs. If I write the number as 10/10, it means 10 reps on one side, followed by 10 reps on the other side. Your body needs to stay balanced!

Day 1: Full Body

This first workout includes some of the best classic body weight exercises to get your sexy self just a li'l bit more sexy.

1. Jump squat × 20 (see page 172)

2. Push-up × 10 (see page 206)

3. Competition burpee × 20 (see page 190)

4. Jump lunge × 10 (see page 173)

5. Mountain climber × 20 (see page 194)

Day 2: Full Body

Today you're going to try variations of lunges and push-ups. And you're going to love it.

1. Side jump lunge × 20 (see page 174)

2. Commando push-up × 12 (see page 208)

3. Prisoner get-up × 12 (see page 188)

4. Split jump × 10 (see page 209)

5. Bird dog × 10 (see page 210)

Day 3: Full Body

Another day to get rid of just a little bit more excess fat. Notice: *excess*. Get to it, guys! Beat your personal best from Day 1!

1. Jump squat × 20 (see page 172)
2. Push-up × 10 (see page 206)
3. Competition burpee × 20 (see page 190)
4. Jump lunge × 10 (see page 173)
5. Mountain climber × 20 (see page 194)

Day 4: Abs

Maybe abs are made in the kitchen, but you need to train them, too! Drop and get that beach body!

1. Plank jack × 20 (see page 211)
2. Flying burpee × 10 (see page 212)
3. Knee hug × 20 (see page 214)
4. Jump tuck × 10 (see page 175)

Day 5: Full Body

Forget the beach body—today we start getting that healthy-for-life body. Beat your personal best from Day 2!

1. Side jump lunge × 20 (see page 174)
2. Commando push-up × 12 (see page 208)
3. Prisoner get-up × 12 (see page 188)

4. Split jump × 10 (see page 209)

5. Bird dog × 10 (see page 210)

Day 6: Lower Body

YAAAA! Buns and thighs!

1. Backward lunge kick-up × 10/10 (see page 184)

2. Sumo jump squat leg lift × 20 alt. (see page 176)

3. Pistol squat to deadlift × 10 alt. (see page 178)

4. Curtsy lunge side kick × 10/10 (see page 179)

5. Squat to lunge jump × 10 (see page 182)

Day 7: Abs

One week hotter. Now annihilate those abdominals, you friggin' fox. Beat your personal best from Day 4!

1. Plank jack × 20 (see page 211)

2. Flying burpee × 10 (see page 212)

3. Knee hug × 20 (see page 214)

4. Jump tuck × 10 (see page 175)

Day 8: Full Body

This workout won't have you jumping for joy—but jumping for a smaller jean size.

1. Regular burpee × 10 (see page 192)

2. Pistol squat × 10 alt. (see page 204)

3. Everest climber × 20 (see page 195)

4. Side-to-side jump × 20 (see page 181)

5. Ab splitters × 10 (see page 217)

Day 9: Lower Body

We're out here trying to get that booty. Keep it up, y'all. Beat your personal best from Day 6!

1. Backward lunge kick-up × 10/10 (see page 184)

2. Sumo jump squat leg lift × 20 alt. (see page 176)

3. Pistol squat × 10 alt. (see page 204)

4. Curtsy lunge side kick × 10/10 (see page 179)

5. Squat to lunge jump × 10 (see page 182)

Day 10: Upper Body

Those guns aren't gonna sculpt themselves. Get to carving!

1. Side burpee × 10 alt. (see page 196)

2. Kick-through push-up × 10 (see page 219)

3. Competition burpee × 10 (see page 190)

4. Plank side jump × 20 (see page 201)

5. Clapping push-up × 5 (see page 202)

Day 11: Full Body

Over one-third of the way done! Kick it up a notch this next third of the plan. Beat your personal best from Day 8, guys!

1. Regular burpee × 10 (see page 192)
2. Pistol squat side kick × 10 alt. (see page 215)
3. Everest climber × 20 (see page 195)
4. Side-to-side jump × 20 (see page 181)
5. Ab splitter × 10 (see page 217)

Day 12: Cardio and Abs

This abdominal workout hits them from all angles for complete development.

1. High knees × 20 (see page 221)
2. Everest climber × 20 (see page 195)
3. Surfer × 20 (see page 200)
4. Competition burpee jump tuck × 10 (see page 191)
5. Side crunch × 10/10 (see page 222)

Day 13: Upper Body

Train for the sleeveless shirts and swimsuit you've been dying to wear! Give today your all. Beat your personal best from Day 10, OK?

1. Side burpee × 10 alt. (see page 196)
2. Kick-through push-up × 10 (see page 219)
3. Competition burpee × 10 (see page 190)

4. Plank side jump × 20 (see page 201)

5. Clapping push-up × 5 (see page 202)

Day 14: Full Body

We're going to increase the challenge now. Stay strong and keep finishing through!

1. Roll back to pistol × 10 alt. (see page 223)

2. Competition burpee to rock-star jump × 10 (see page 224)

3. Dive-bomber push-up × 10 (see page 225)

4. Crab toe touch × 20 (see page 227)

5. Pike press to jump tuck × 10 (see page 228)

Day 15: Cardio and Abs

Beat your personal best from Day 12! People with fitness goals succeed when they know where they're going. Let's see some purpose today!

1. High knees × 20 (see page 221)

2. Everest climber × 20 (see page 195)

3. Surfer × 20 (see page 200)

4. Competition burpee jump tuck × 10 (see page 191)

5. Side crunch × 10/10 (see page 222)

Day 16: Lower Body

These combo moves really crank up the calorie burning!

1. Surrender squat to front kick × 10/10 (see page 187)

2. Jump tuck to pistol × 10 alt. (see page 230)

3. Push-up jump to squat × 10 (see page 199)

4. One-leg deadlift to front kick × 10/10 (see page 231)

5. Backward lunge jump-up × 10/10 (see page 180)

Day 17: Full Body

Another day, another opportunity. Make this the best one yet.

1. Roll back to pistol × 10 alt. (see page 223)

2. Competition burpee to rock-star jump × 10 (see page 224)

3. Dive-bomber push-up × 10 (see page 225)

4. Crab toe touch × 20 (see page 227)

5. Pike press to jump tuck × 10 (see page 228)

Day 18: Upper Body

The moves are becoming harder, but you're becoming tougher. And hotter. (We know, we didn't think it was possible either.)

1. Push-up to one-leg jump-up × 10 alt. (see page 232)

2. One-arm press-up × 10/10 (see page 234)

3. Pike press to jump tuck × 10 (see page 228)

4. Twisted push-up toe touch × 10 alt. (see page 235)

5. Knee hug × 20 (see page 214)

Day 19: Lower Body

Bye-bye, Cellulite Sally! Hello, Miss Daisy Duke. Beat your personal best from Day 16!

1. Surrender squat to front kick × 10/10 (see page 187)

2. Jump tuck to pistol × 10 alt. (see page 230)

3. Push-up jump to squat × 10 (see page 199)

4. One-leg deadlift to front kick × 10/10 (see page 231)

5. Backward lunge jump-up × 10/10 (see page 180)

Day 20: Full Body

Start strong, finish strong, and kick butt in between.

1. Jump lunge × 20 (see page 173)

2. Flying burpee × 10 (see page 212)

3. Ab splitters × 10 (see page 217)

4. Pistol squat side kick × 10 alt. (see page 215)

5. Clapping push-up × 5 (see page 202)

6. Surfer × 20 (see page 200)

Day 21: Upper Body

Beat your personal best from Day 18, guys! You already have the perfect body. Now you just have to find it.

1. Push-up to one-leg jump-up × 10 alt. (see page 232)

2. One-arm press-up × 10/10 (see page 234)

3. Pike press to jump tuck × 10 (see page 228)

4. Twisted push-up toe touch × 10 alt. (see page 235)

5. Knee hugs × 20 (see page 214)

Day 22: Cardio and Abs

The end is near, my friends! Keep going so your end is looking right by then!

1. Competition burpee jump tuck × 10 (see page 191)

2. Side crunch × 10/10 (see page 222)

3. Split jump × 10 (see page 209)

4. Plank jack × 20 (see page 211)

5. Knee hug × 20 (see page 214)

6. Push-up jump to squat × 10 (see page 199)

Day 23: Full Body

This is one of my all-time favorite workouts!

1. Jump lunge × 20 (see page 173)

2. Flying burpee × 10 (see page 212)

3. Ab splitter × 10 (see page 217)

4. Side jump lunge × 20 (see page 174)

5. Clapping push-up × 5 (see page 202)

6. Surfer × 20 (see page 200)

Day 24: Full Body

Only six more days! Try to incorporate these workouts even after the plan is over.

1. Jump squat × 20 (see page 172)

2. Santana push-up × 10 alt. sides (see page 198)

3. Pistol squat × 10 alt. legs (see page 204)

4. Commando push-up × 10 alt. legs (see page 208)

5. Sumo jump squat leg lift × 20 alt. legs (see page 176)

6. Bird dog × 10 alt. (see page 210)

Day 25: Cardio and Abs

Beat your personal best from Day 22! Sore or sorry? The choice is yours.

1. Competition burpee jump tuck × 10 (see page 191)

2. Side crunch × 10/10 (see page 222)

3. Split jump × 10 (see page 209)

4. Plank jack × 20 (see page 211)

5. Knee hug × 20 (see page 214)

6. Push-up jump to squat × 10 (see page 199)

Day 26: Lower Body

Nice butt.

1. Backward lunge jump-up × 10/10 (see page 180)

2. Jump squat × 20 (see page 172)

3. Surrender squat to front kick × 10/10 (see page 187)

4. Side-to-side jump × 20 (see page 181)

5. Crossed-leg jump squat toe touch × 20 alt. (see page 185)

6. Curtsy lunge side kick × 10/10 (see page 179)

Day 27: Full Body

We at it again! All over. Feel the buuuuurn. Beat your personal best from Day 24!

1. Jump squat × 20 (see page 172)

2. Santana push-up × 10 alt. sides (see page 198)

3. Sumo squat leg lift × 10 alt. legs (see page 237)

4. Commando push-up × 10 alt. legs (see page 208)

5. Sumo jump squat leg lift × 20 alt. legs (see page 176)

6. Bird dog × 10 alt. (see page 210)

Day 28: Full Body

Make today's workout as solid as your biceps. Yeah. Solid as a rock.

1. Rock-star jump × 20 (see page 238)

2. Dive-bomber push-up × 10 (see page 225)

3. Roll back to pistol × 10 alt. (see page 223)

4. Squat to lunge jump × 10 (see page 182)

5. Everest climber × 20 (see page 195)

6. Prisoner get-up × 10 (see page 188)

Day 29: Lower Body

You never know how much you want something until it comes to putting in the work. Beat your personal best from Day 26!

1. Backward lunge jump-up × 10/10 (see page 180)

2. Jump squat × 20 (see page 172)

3. Surrender squat to front kick × 10/10 (see page 187)

4. Side-to-side jump × 20 (see page 181)

5. Crossed-leg jump squat toe touch × 20 alt. (see page 185)

6. Curtsy lunge side kick × 10/10 (see page 179)

Day 30: Full Body

We goin' in! Last day! Demolish this workout and then look how far you've come! Beat your personal best from Day 28, guys!

1. Rock-star jump × 20 (see page 238)

2. Dive-bomber push-up × 10 (see page 225)

3. Roll back to pistol × 10 alt. (see page 223)

4. Squat to lunge jump × 10 (see page 182)

5. Everest climber × 20 (see page 195)

6. Prisoner get-up × 10 (see page 188)

Exercise Descriptions

1. JUMP SQUAT

Starting position: Feet shoulder-width apart, standing tall.

Movement: Push your hips back, keeping your back straight, and descend until your thighs are parallel to the ground. Then push off your heels and use the power of your hips to jump up. Land with your feet shoulder-width apart. Repeat for desired number of reps or time allotted.

Be careful to: Brace your abs to support your core and keep your shoulders back and down.

Notes: No part of your body should be relaxed at any point during a jump squat.

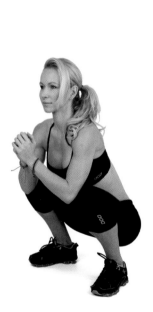
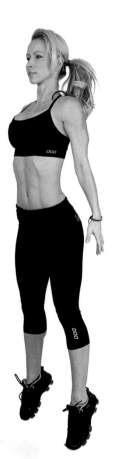

2. JUMP LUNGE

Starting position: Front leg in a 90-degree angle, knee pointing straight forward just like your toes. Back knee just a few inches off the ground.

Movement: Using the power of your hips, jump up and switch legs. Continue in alternating fashion.

Be careful to: Brace your abs and keep your chest up.

Notes: An easier variation of these would be scissors, when you don't need to go as low into the lunge and your knees are only slightly bent.

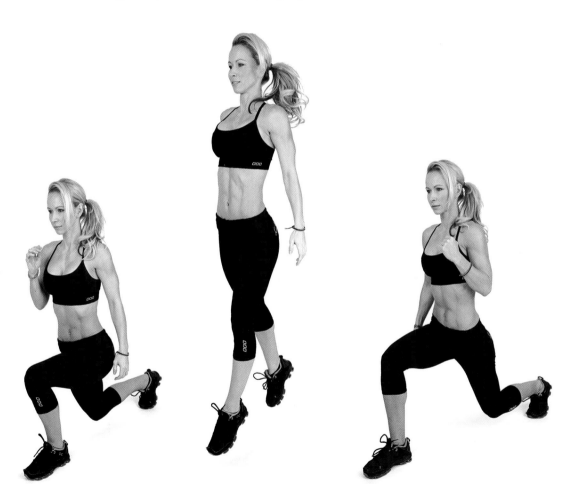

3. SIDE JUMP LUNGE

Starting position: Feet wide apart, weight shifted toward your right leg. Left leg fully extended to the side, left foot flat on the ground.

Movement: Squat and touch the ground with your left hand before pushing off your right foot to jump up and switch legs. Continue in alternating fashion.

Be careful to: Keep your back straight when you push your hips back.

Notes: Make sure your right knee is pointing straight forward just like your right toes.

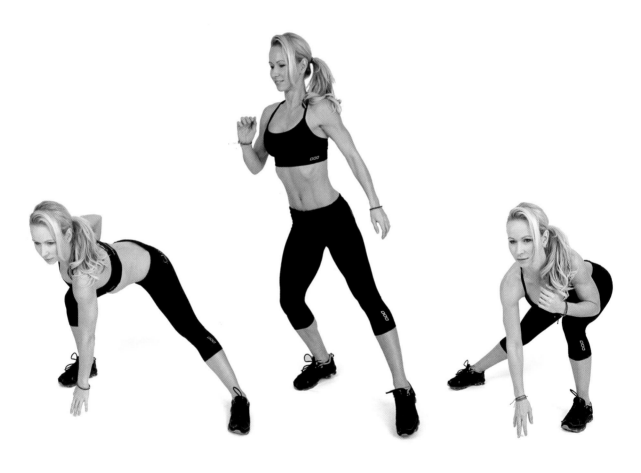

4. JUMP TUCK

Starting position: Low squat position.

Movement: Jump as high as you can and tuck your knees toward your chest.

Be careful to: Land softly on the balls of your feet.

Notes: Bring your knees as close to your chest as possible at the top.

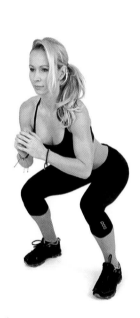
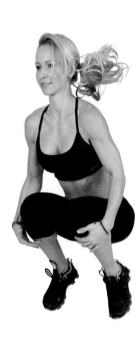

5. SUMO JUMP SQUAT LEG LIFT

Starting position: Feet wide apart, toes pointing slightly outward. Knees are pointing the same direction as your feet. Bend your knees and push your hips back until your thighs are parallel to the ground.

Movement: Jump up, and as you land in the starting position, shift your weight immediately toward one leg and lift the other leg out to the side.

Be careful to: Land softly on the balls of your feet.

Notes: Alternate legs on each jump.

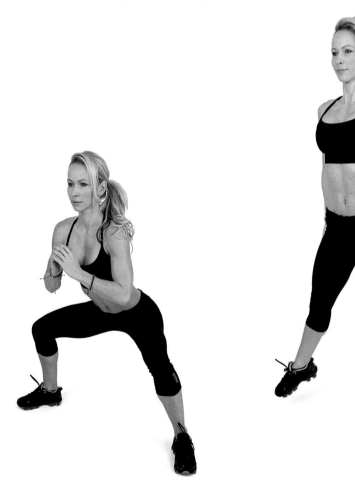

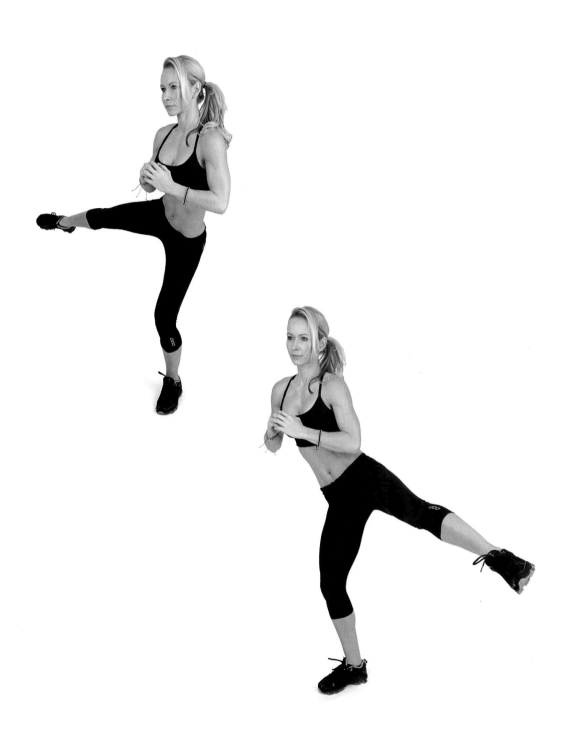

6. PISTOL SQUAT TO DEADLIFT

Starting position: Standing tall, chest up, shoulders back. Extend your left leg and your arms in front of you and brace your abs.

Movement: Tense all the muscles in the standing leg and squat all the way down. Your weight should be mostly on your heel. Pushing off of the heel, stand up and squeeze your glutes as you push your hips forward. From there, bend at the waist to lower your torso toward the floor, lifting your left leg behind you. Straighten back up, still on the one leg.

Be careful to: If you find yourself wobbling in the top position, you need to really tense all the muscles in the standing leg.

Notes: Do the same number of reps on each side. The pistol modification (page 205) is for those of you who find the regular pistol squat intimidating.

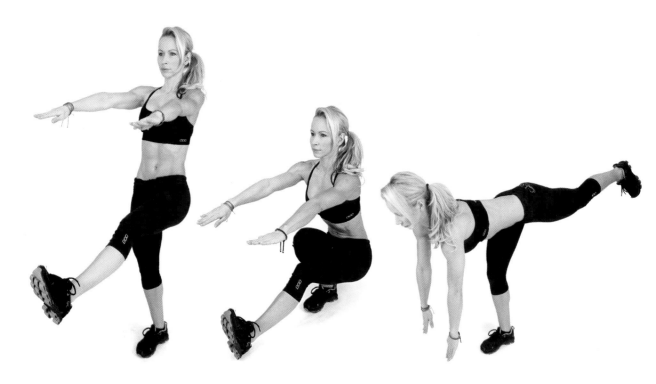

7. CURTSY LUNGE SIDE KICK

Starting position: Standing tall.

Movement: Take a deep step back and to the side with your right leg so that it extends across and behind your left leg. Bring your right knee down to the ground and then push off your left leg. As you stand back up, kick your right leg out to the side.

Be careful to: Avoid hyperextending your knee joint when kicking out your leg.

Notes: Alternate legs or do the same number of reps on each leg. You can modify this exercise and do a leg lift instead of a kick.

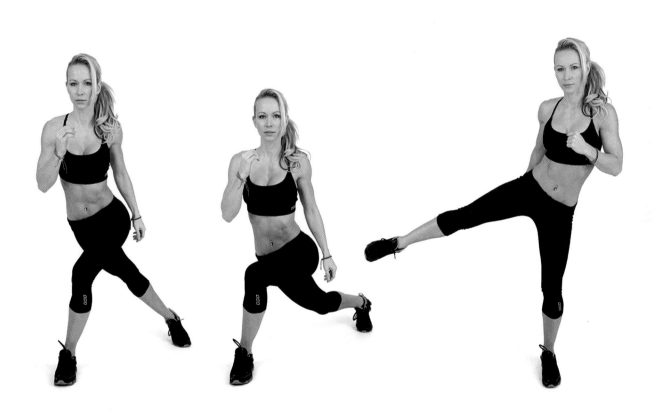

8. BACKWARD LUNGE JUMP-UP

Starting position: Standing tall.

Movement: Take a deep step back with your right leg and drop your hips so that your right knee touches the ground. Push off your left foot to jump up, bringing your right knee up in front of you. Land softly on the ball of your left foot and drop right back into the lunge position.

Be careful to: Keep your chest up while dropping into the lunge.

Notes: Do all of your reps for one leg before switching to the other.

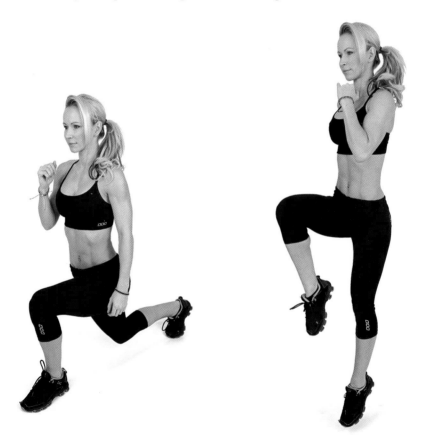

Modification: An easier modification of this exercise would be just the knee up without the jump.

9. SIDE-TO-SIDE JUMP

Starting position: Standing tall with your feet together.

Movement: Jump sideways over a small obstacle such as a book or a yoga block. Continue jumping back and forth.

Be careful to: Keep your abs engaged throughout the exercise.

Notes: This is a great cardio exercise if you do all the reps as fast as you can.

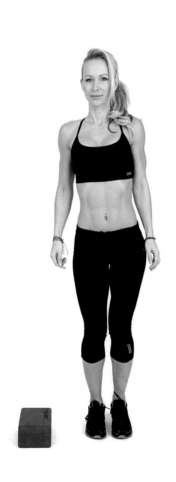
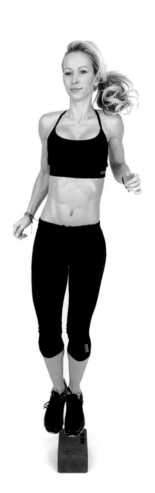

10. SQUAT TO LUNGE JUMP

Starting position: Low squat. Hips back until your thighs are parallel to the ground.

Movement: Jump! In the air, bring your left leg forward and your right leg back so that you land in a lunge position. Jump out of the lunge and right back into the squat. Jump up again, this time with your right leg forward and left leg back. Jump back into the squat.

Be careful to: Keep your back straight during the squatting portion of this exercise.

Notes: Jumping in and out of lunge counts as one rep. Make sure you're always alternating legs.

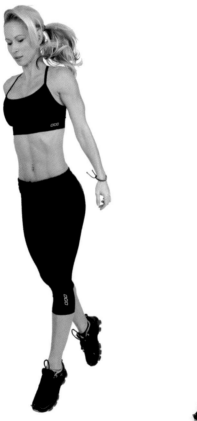
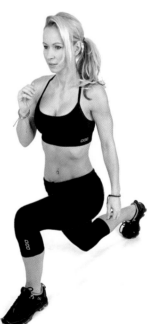

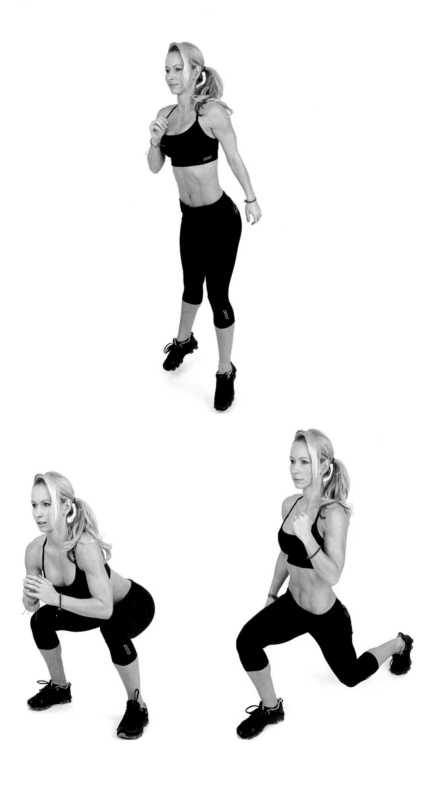

11. BACKWARD LUNGE KICK-UP

Starting position: Standing tall.

Movement: Take a large step back into lunge position with your front knee and toes pointing straight forward. Push off your front foot to stand up and kick the back leg as high up in front of you as possible. Return into the lunge position.

Be careful to: Keep your chest up and shoulders back and down throughout the movement.

Notes: Always do the same number of reps for both legs.

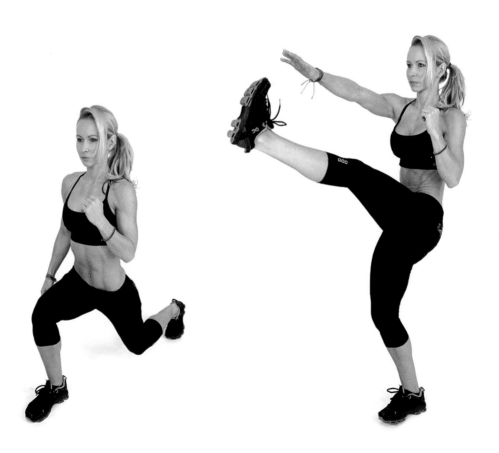

12. CROSSED-LEG JUMP SQUAT TOE TOUCH

Starting position: Standing tall, arms at your sides, feet shoulder-width apart.

Movement: Jump and then land with your left foot crisscrossed behind your right, letting your knees give a little as you land. Immediately jump again, this time bringing your legs apart in a wide stance. As you land, squat and reach across your body with your left hand to touch your right foot. Immediately jump again, this time crisscrossing your right foot behind your left. As you land, squat and reach across your body with your right hand to touch your left foot. Continue in alternating fashion.

Be careful to: Make sure your back is not rounding during the squat.

Notes: This exercise combo should be done fast so that each movement flows into the next one.

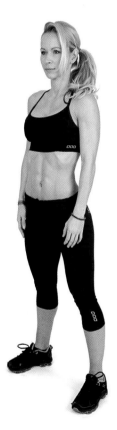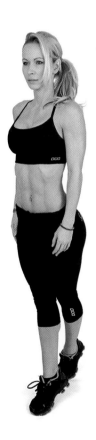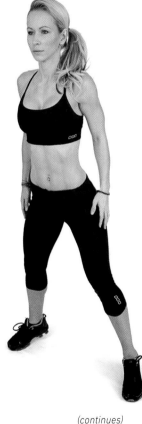

(continues)

Crossed-Leg Jump Squat Toe Touch (continued)

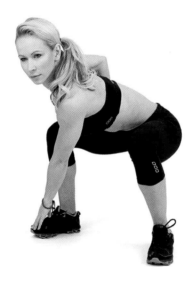
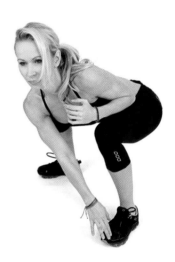

13. SURRENDER SQUAT TO FRONT KICK

Starting position: Standing on your right leg, tensing all of the muscles including your glutes and abs.

Movement: Squat all the way down on your right leg until you bring your left knee on the ground and sit on your left heel. Pushing off your right heel to stand up, kick your left leg up in front of you.

Be careful to: Focus on not rounding your back during the squat.

Notes: Always do the same number of reps per side.

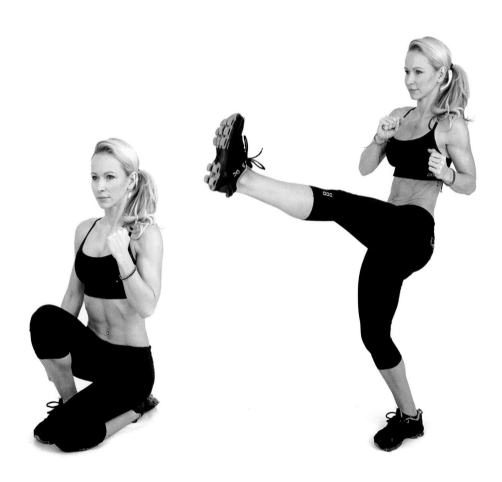

14. PRISONER GET-UP

Starting position: Lying on your back with your hands clasped behind your head.

Movement: Bring your left foot underneath your right knee and plant your right foot firmly on the ground. Crunch your abs and do a sit-up, Pushing off your right foot, get your left knee on the ground for support. Pushing off your right heel, stand all the way up. Now reverse the movement and return to the ground the same way you got up.

Be careful to: Focus on not rounding your back.

Modification: If this move is too difficult, get your left foot rather than your left knee on the ground for support. Make sure you switch legs after each rep and complete an equal number for both.

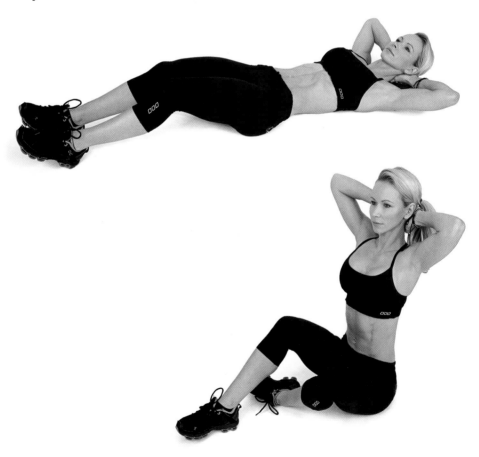

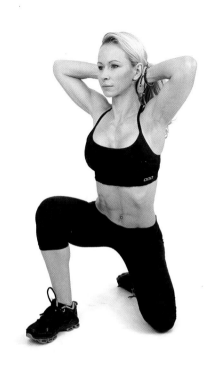

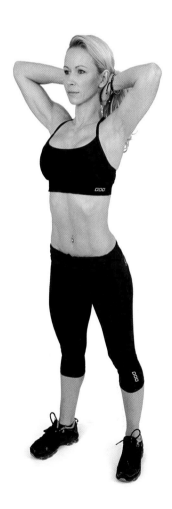

15. COMPETITION BURPEE

Starting position: Standing tall.

Movement: Drop down until your chest touches the floor. Push yourself off the floor and jump your feet forward into a squat. Then jump up as high as you can before returning to the ground or floor.

Be careful to: Be quick—but don't hurry.

Notes: To make this slightly harder, clap your hands at the top.

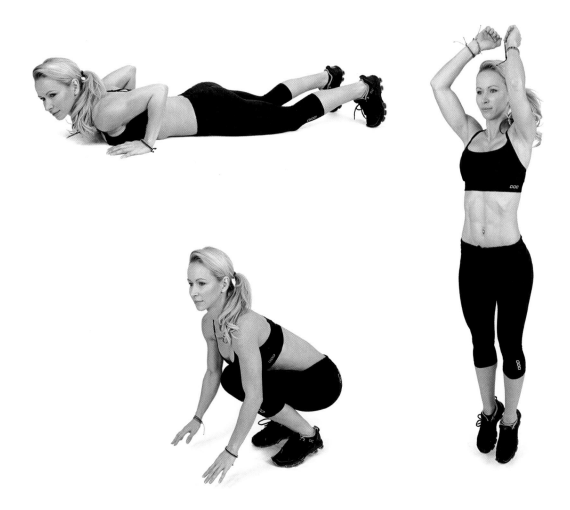

16. COMPETITION BURPEE JUMP TUCK

Starting position: Standing tall.

Movement: Drop down until your chest touches the floor. Push yourself off the floor and jump your feet forward into a squat. Then jump up as high as you can while tucking your knees in toward your chest. Return to the ground or floor.

Be careful to: Be quick—but don't hurry.

Notes: To make this slightly harder, clap your hands at the top.

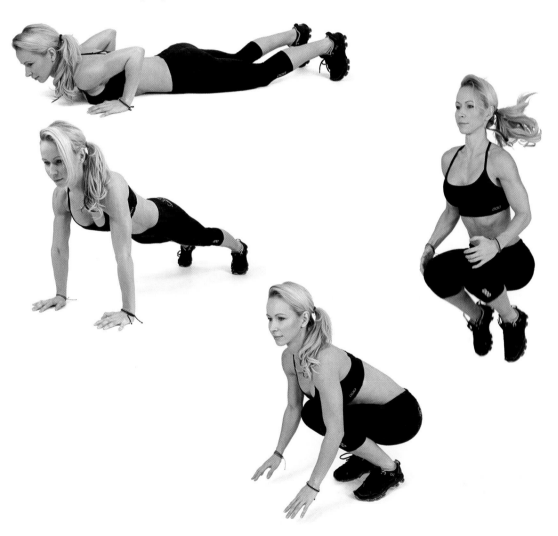

17. REGULAR BURPEE

Starting position: A basic push-up position, with your hands directly underneath your shoulders and your body in a straight line. Make sure not to drop your hips or push them up. Tense all the muscles in your body, including your legs, glutes, and abs.

Movement: Bend your elbows to lower your body as close to the ground as possible. Push up and then jump your feet forward into a squat. Jump up as high as you can. Return to the ground or floor.

Be careful to: Keep your elbows from flaring out during the push-up portion.

Notes: An easier variation of this exercise would be the competition burpee (page 190).

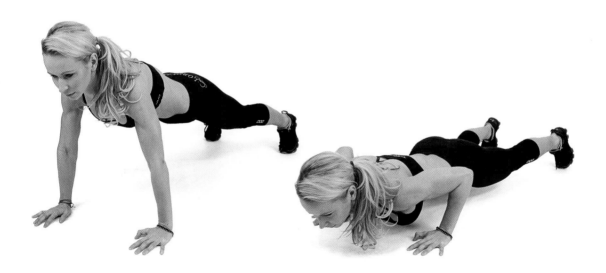

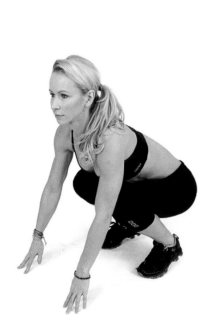

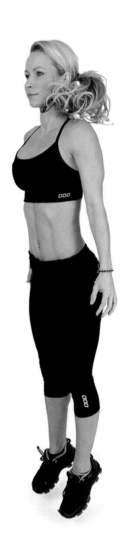

18. MOUNTAIN CLIMBER

Starting position: A basic push-up position, with your hands directly underneath your shoulders and your body in a straight line. Tense all the muscles in your body, including your legs, glutes, and abs.

Movement: Bring one knee forward as far as you can. Jump, switch legs, and repeat.

Be careful to: Your feet should land at the same time.

Notes: The movement should primarily occur in the hips. Your torso shouldn't move much at all.

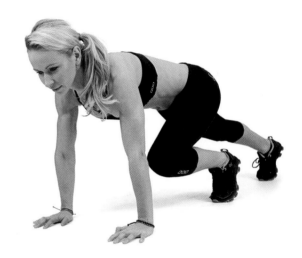

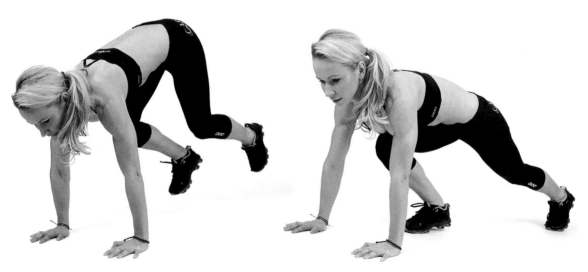

19. EVEREST CLIMBER

Starting position: A basic push-up position, with your hands directly underneath your shoulders and your body in a straight line. Make sure not to drop your hips or push them up. Tense all the muscles in your body, including your legs, glutes, and abs.

Movement: Take a large step forward with your left foot right next to your left hand. Now jump and switch legs. Continue in alternating fashion.

Be careful to: Be warmed up before you attempt this, as this exercise requires a lot of flexibility and mobility.

Notes: An easier variation of this exercise would be the mountain climber (opposite).

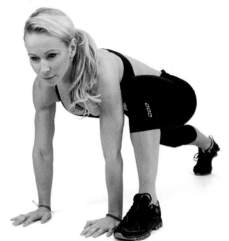

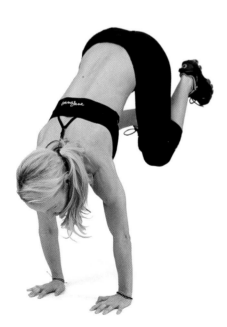

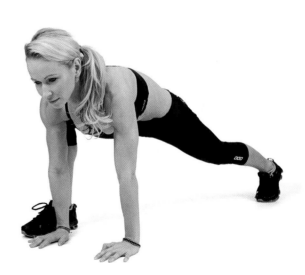

20. SIDE BURPEE

Starting position: Standing tall.

Movement: Squat down, put your hands on the ground off to one side shoulder-width apart, fingertips pointing to each other, and jump both feet to the opposite side. Then do a push-up. Jump your feet forward again into a squat and then jump up. Alternate sides.

Be careful to: Try not to drop your hips. Reach for the ceiling on your jump.

Modification: If you're a beginner, you can step rather than jump to the side. Make sure to do the same number of reps on both sides.

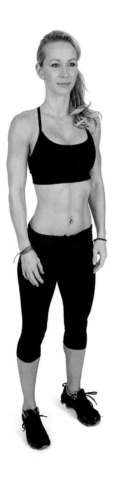
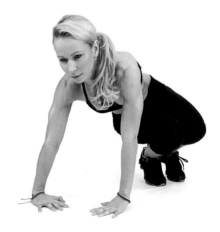

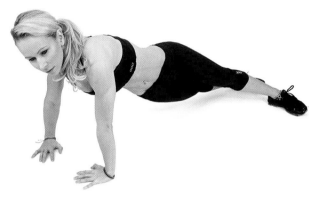

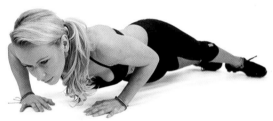

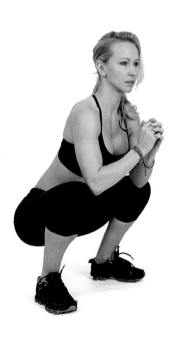

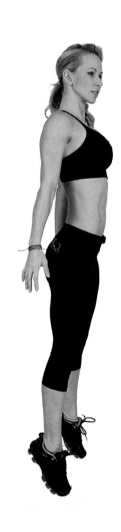

21. SANTANA PUSH-UP

Starting position: A basic push-up position, with your hands directly underneath your shoulders and your body in a straight line. Make sure not to drop your hips or push them up. Tense all the muscles in your body, including your legs, glutes, and abs.

Movement: Bend your elbows to lower your torso toward the floor. Push back up to the top position and then lift one arm all the way toward the ceiling, keeping your eyes on the hand and twisting your torso along with your arm.

Be careful to: Make sure you're not dropping your hips when raising your arm.

Notes: Alternate or do one side at a time; either way, do the same number of reps on each side.

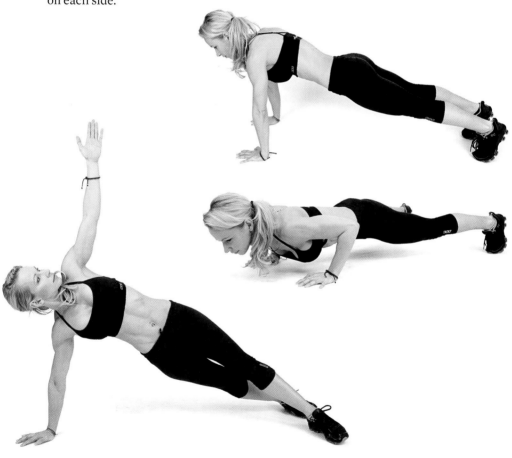

22. PUSH-UP JUMP TO SQUAT

Starting position: A basic push-up position, with your hands directly underneath your shoulders and your body in a straight line. Make sure not to drop your hips or push them up. Tense all the muscles in your body, including your legs, glutes, and abs.

Movement: Bend your elbows and lower your torso until it nearly touches the ground. Press back up. At the top, jump straight into the bottom of a squat position. Chest up, back straight. Your feet should land where your hands were. Unlike a burpee, your hands will leave the ground; it's a more powerful move. Also unlike a burpee, don't jump up out of the squat; from there resume the top of the push-up position.

Be careful to: Keep your elbows from flaring out. Don't drop your hips, and don't push them up either.

Notes: Make sure your body is tight in the push-up position.

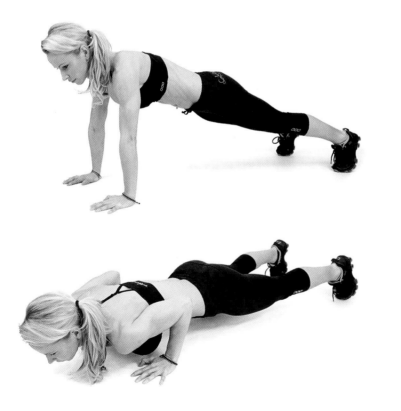

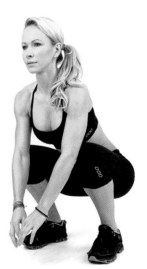

23. SURFER

Starting position: Flat on your belly, hands flat on the ground under your shoulders.

Movement: Push off the ground and jump right up, with feet spread wide and your weight on your heels. Imagine you're on a surfboard and you need to keep one leg back and one leg forward. Drop down onto your belly and power up again.

Be careful to: Stay balanced throughout the movement, like a surfer catching a wave.

Notes: Switch legs for each rep and make sure you're pushing your hips back and keeping your back straight.

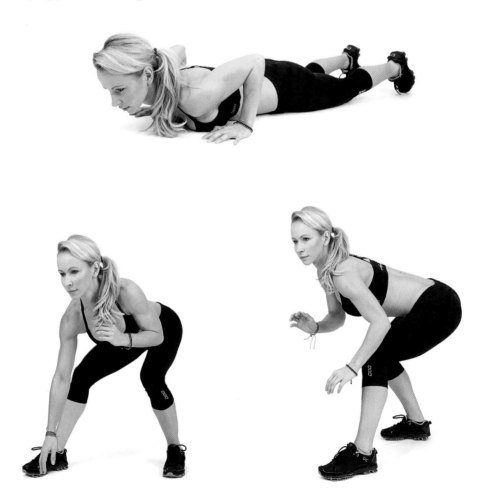

24. PLANK SIDE JUMP

Starting position: A basic push-up position, with your hands directly underneath your shoulders and your body in a straight line. Make sure not to drop your hips or push them up. Tense all the muscles in your body, including your legs, glutes, and abs.

Movement: Jump forward and out to the side with your feet together. Jump back into the top of the push-up position and then jump with your feet forward toward the other side.

Be careful to: Don't drop your hips, and don't push them up either.

Notes: Maintain a tight core throughout the movement.

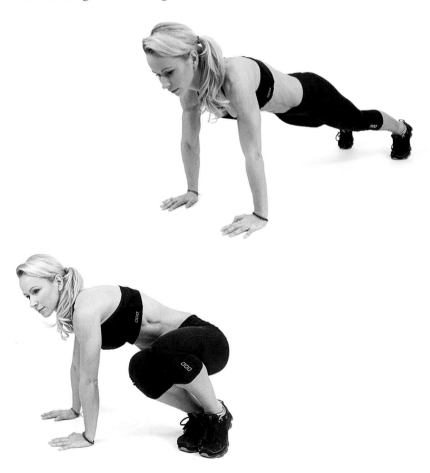

25. CLAPPING PUSH-UP

Starting position: A basic push-up position, with your hands directly underneath your shoulders and your body in a straight line. Make sure not to drop your hips or push them up. Tense all the muscles in your body, including your legs, glutes, and abs.

Movement: Bend your elbows halfway down to the ground or floor and then use all your power to push yourself off the ground and clap your hands together. Stabilize in the top position for a second and then start another rep.

Be careful to: Don't drop your hips and don't push them up either.

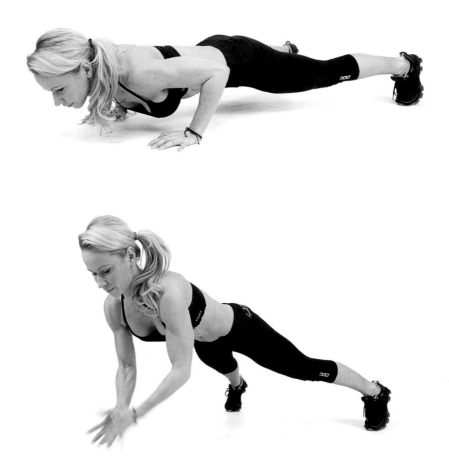

Modification: Try tensing all of your muscles throughout the exercise. If that's too hard, try this easier modification. Get down onto your hands and knees and cross your ankles. Push your pelvis forward so that your body is in one line from your shoulders to your knees. Do your best not to stick your butt out and focus on engaging your abs. Bend your elbows and bring your body close to the ground. Push off the ground with a lot of power and clap your hands together.

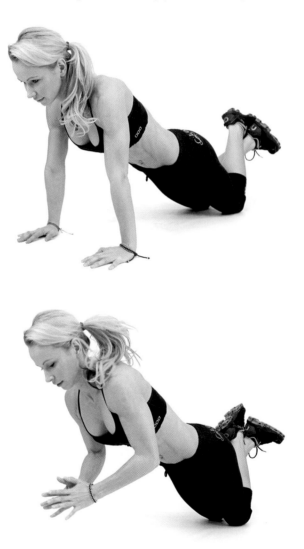

26. PISTOL SQUAT

Starting position: Standing tall, chest up, shoulders back and down. Extend your left leg and your arms in front of you and brace your abs.

Movement: Tense all of the muscles in the standing leg and squat all the way down, keeping your left leg extended out in front of you. At the bottom, your weight should be mostly on your right heel and your left leg should be parallel to the floor. Pushing off your right heel, stand up and squeeze your glutes as you push your hips forward to return to standing.

Be careful to: If you find yourself wobbling in the top position, you need to really tense all of the muscles in the standing leg.

Notes: Do the same number of reps for each side.

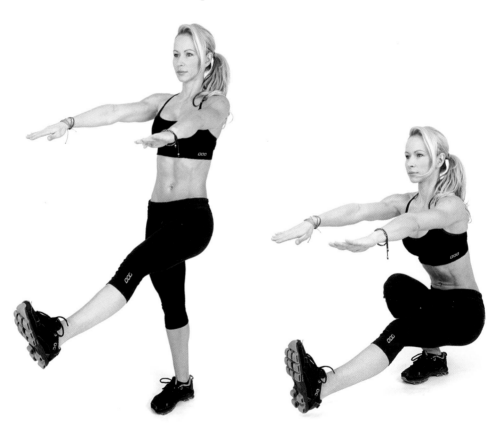

Modification: If you find pistol squats intimidating or if you don't yet have the flexibility necessary to go all the way down to the floor, then put a stool or low chair behind you and squat down till your butt touches the chair, then stand up.

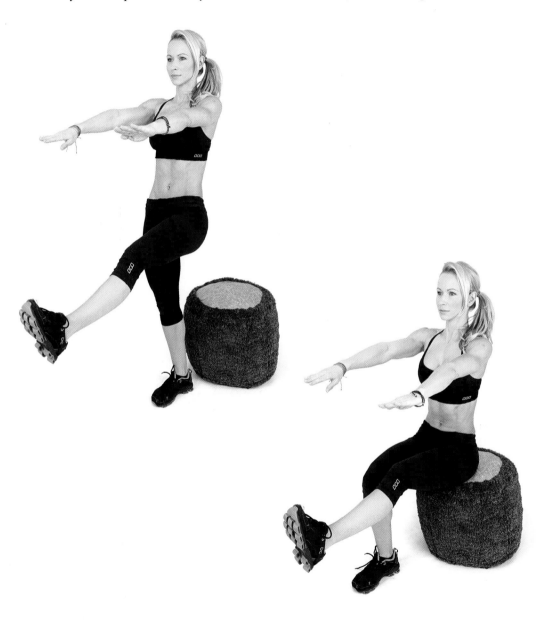

27. PUSH-UP

Starting position: A basic push-up position, with your hands directly underneath your shoulders and your body in a straight line. Make sure not to drop your hips or push them up. Tense all the muscles in your body, including your legs, glutes, and abs.

Movement: Bend your elbows and lower your torso until your chest almost touches the floor. Straighten your arms to press your torso back up to the starting position.

Be careful to: Keep your elbows from flaring. Don't drop your hips or arch your back.

Notes: Squeeze your chest as you press your upper body back up to the starting position.

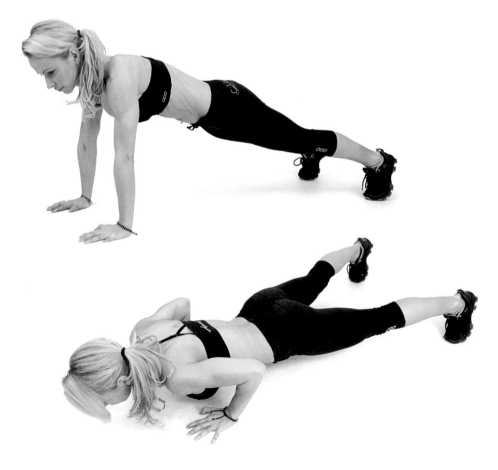

Modification: If a push-up is too difficult, keep your knees on the floor.

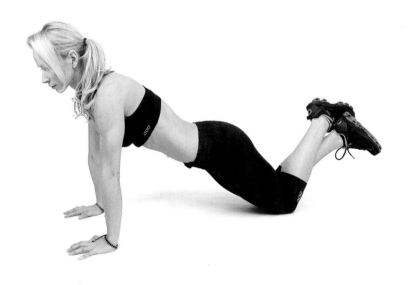

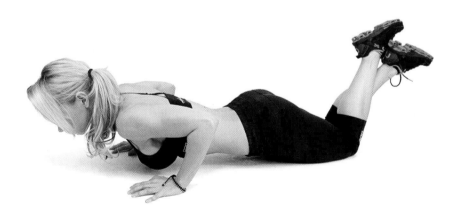

28. COMMANDO PUSH-UP

Starting position: Lying on your belly, hands flat on the floor beneath your shoulders.

The movement: Push down with your hands to raise your torso off the floor. Draw one knee toward your chest and then return it to its starting position before lowering back to the floor. Repeat—only this time tuck the other knee. Return to the floor. Repeat the push-ups and the knee tucks.

Be careful to: Keep the movement tight and focused on your hips when drawing in your knee.

Notes: In the top position, your form should be as tight as if you were doing normal push-ups. Don't get sloppy!

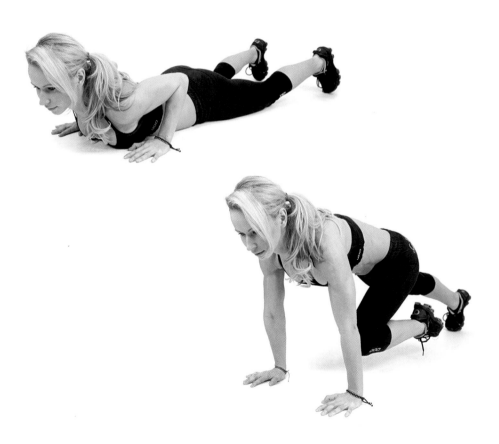

29. SPLIT JUMP

Starting position: Standing, feet planted and hands at your sides.

Movement: Descend into a body weight squat. At the bottom, jump as high as you can, bending your knees and scissoring your legs so that one foot travels in front of you and one trails behind you. Land with your feet in the starting position.

Be careful to: Absorb the impact upon landing; don't be too rigid.

Notes: Continue jumping in alternating fashion for the duration of the set, so that for the next rep, the leg that trailed now leads, and vice versa.

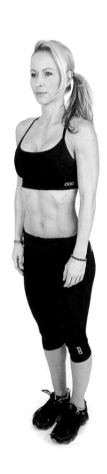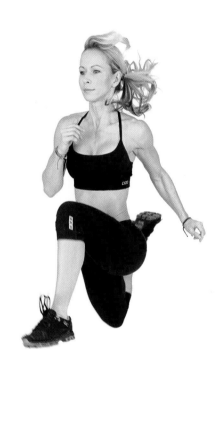

30. BIRD DOG

Starting position: Top of a push-up.

Movement: Lift one leg up and point it directly out behind you; take the opposing arm and reach directly out in front of you. Hold this position for several seconds. Return to the starting position and extend the other leg behind you; take the opposing arm and reach directly out in front of you. Hold this position for several seconds.

Be careful to: Brace your abs so your torso stays flat; don't let it sag or arch.

Notes: Continue alternating for the desired number of reps or the time allotted.

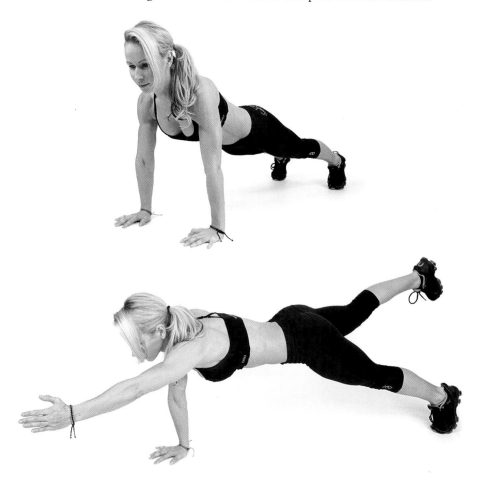

31. PLANK JACK

Starting position: A basic push-up position, with your hands directly underneath your shoulders and your body in a straight line. Make sure not to drop your hips or push them up. Tense all the muscles in your body, including your legs, glutes, and abs.

Movement: Jump your feet apart so your lower body forms a V after you land on your toes. Then bring your feet back together.

Be careful to: Keep your abs tight throughout the movement.

Notes: Continue for the desired number of reps or the time allotted.

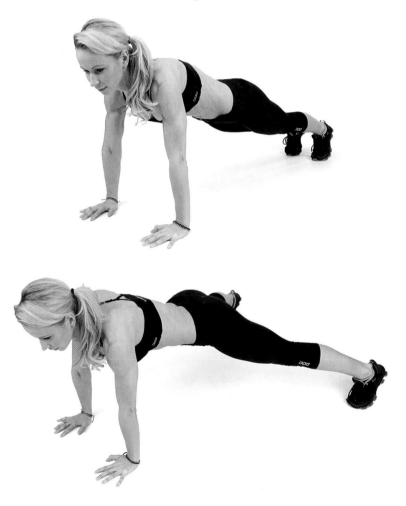

32. FLYING BURPEE

Starting position: Standing in front of your exercise mat, feet shoulder-width apart, hips dropped back behind you so that you're in a chair pose, ideally with your thighs parallel to the ground. Your back should be angled but straight and your core tight.

Movement: Drop your butt down onto the mat and then raise your legs into the air in a hip thrust. Roll forward into a push-up position and immediately do a push-up. Jump up into a burpee and then return to the chair position from which you started.

Be careful to: Keep your back straight each time you return to the starting position.

Notes: It's hard, but this is one of my favorite exercises.

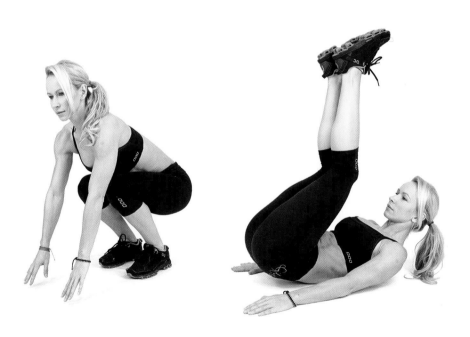

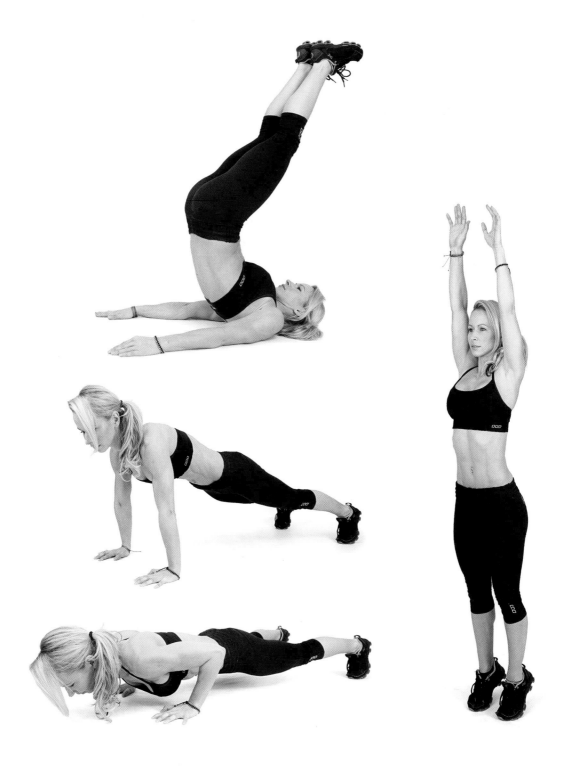

33. KNEE HUG

Starting position: Lie on your back with your legs extended in front of you, slightly off the floor, and your arms at your side.

Movement: Draw your knees in toward your torso and hug them briefly before returning the starting position. Immediately repeat the movement.

Be careful to: Keep your abs tight throughout. Imagine someone is about to punch you in the stomach.

Notes: Continue alternating for the desired number of reps or the time allotted.

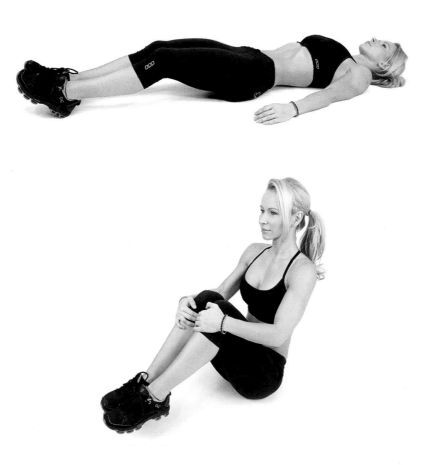

34. PISTOL SQUAT SIDE KICK

Starting position: Stand on one leg and extend the other leg in front of you, tensing all of the muscles in the standing leg, including your glutes. Extend your arms in front of you for balance.

Movement: Bend your hips and knees to squat without rounding your upper back. Get your butt all the way down until it's only inches off the ground. Push off the heel and stand up, pushing your hips forward. Lean your body toward the side of the standing leg and kick the other leg up and out to the side.

Be careful of: Even though you're kicking, the move should still be under control.

Notes: Repeat the same number of reps on each side.

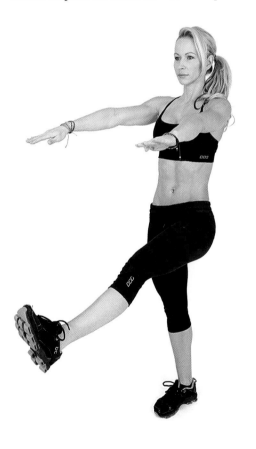

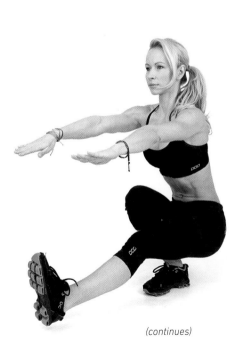

(continues)

Pistol Squat Side Kick *(continued)*

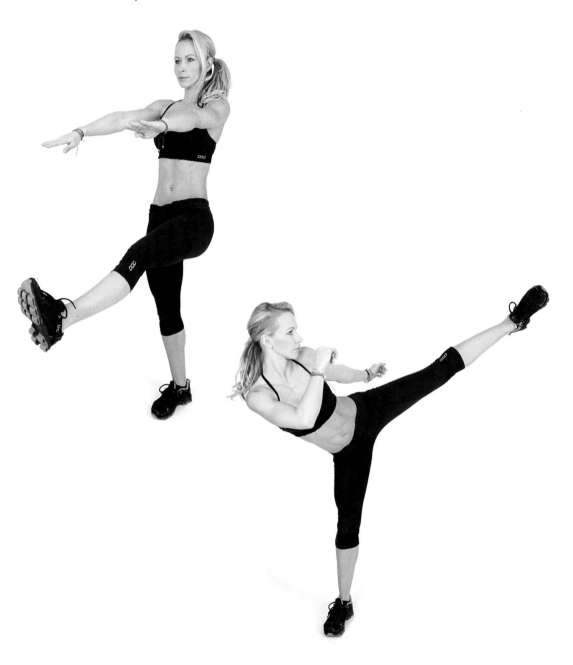

35. AB SPLITTERS

Starting position: Lying on your back with your legs extended in front of you, slightly off the floor, arms at your side.

Movement: Raise your legs up and reach high to touch your toes before briefly returning to the starting position. Immediately scissor-kick your legs out and try to touch the ground by reaching through your open legs. Immediately draw your knees in toward your torso and hug them briefly before returning to the starting position.

Be careful to: Keep your abs tense throughout the movement.

Notes: Continue for the desired number of reps or the time allotted.

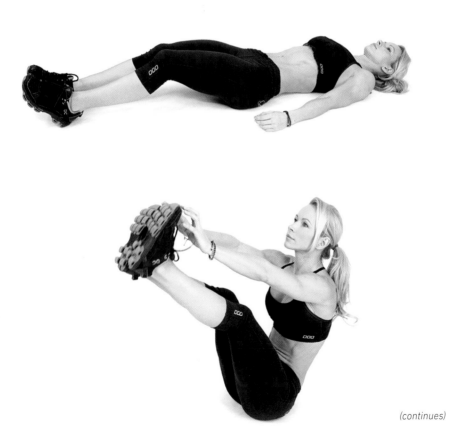

(continues)

Ab Splitters (continued)

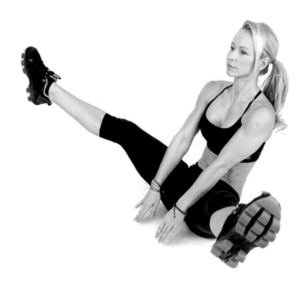

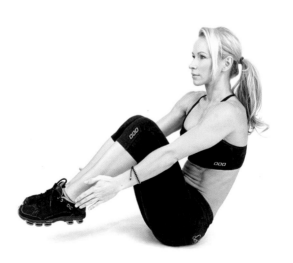

36. KICK-THROUGH PUSH-UP

Starting position: A basic push-up position, with your hands directly underneath your shoulders and your body in a straight line. Make sure not to drop your hips or push them up. Tense all the muscles in your body, including your legs, glutes, and abs.

Movement: Step forward with your left foot until it's next to your left hand, then lift your left hand off the ground and kick your right leg through and in between your right arm and left foot. Return to the starting position and do a push-up. Repeat the movement so that this time you kick your left leg through and in between your left arm and right foot. Continue in alternating fashion.

Be careful to: Stay tight in the push-up position.

Notes: This will challenge the flexibility in your hips. Don't get discouraged!

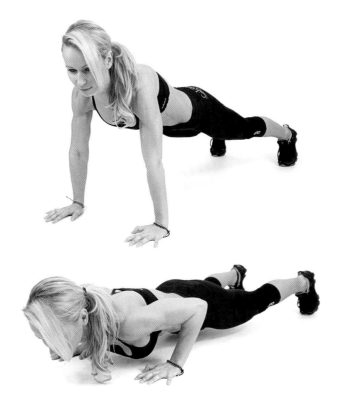

(continues)

Kick-Through Push-Up (continued)

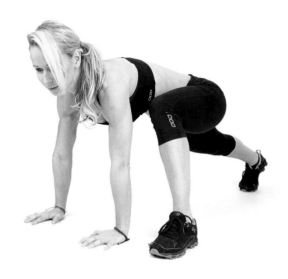

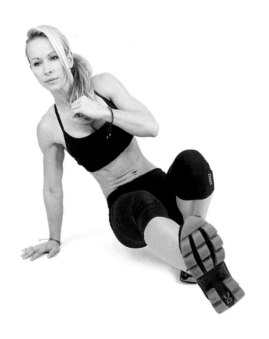

37. HIGH KNEES

Starting position: Standing tall.

Movement: Run in place, bringing your knees as high as possible in exaggerated fashion.

Be careful to: Keep your chest up throughout the movement. Lean your torso slightly back to engage your abs more.

Notes: This move should also improve your running technique.

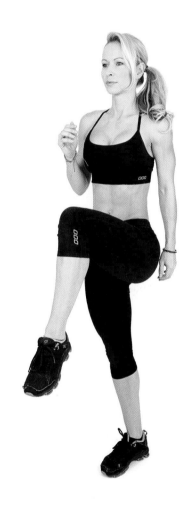

38. SIDE CRUNCH

Starting position: Lying on the floor, legs extended, one hand on the ground, the other behind your head.

Movement: Bring the elbow of the arm/hand behind your head toward your knees in a crunching movement. Lift your legs off the ground so your knees and elbows meet halfway. Return to the starting position.

Be careful to: Not pull on your head with your hand; you'll hurt your neck!

Notes: After completing your reps with that elbow, switch sides and arm positions and do the same number on the other side.

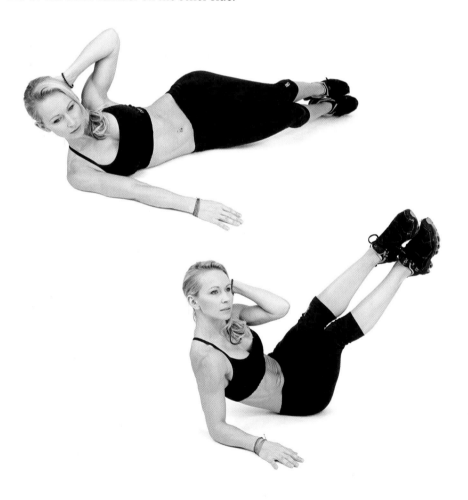

39. ROLL BACK TO PISTOL

Starting position: Standing in front of your mat on one leg, tensing all of the muscles in the standing leg.

Movement: Extend your arms and the other leg in front of you and start pushing your hips back, while keeping your back straight. Squat all the way down until your butt touches the ground and you roll back to bring the extended leg over your head. Use the momentum and roll forward to stand up on the same leg. Push off the heel and use the power of your hips to get back into the standing position. Do the same number of reps using each leg.

Be careful to: Go nice and deep on your squat or you won't benefit fully!

Notes: You can modify this exercise by not extending the other leg in front of you but by keeping your toes lightly on the ground for better balance.

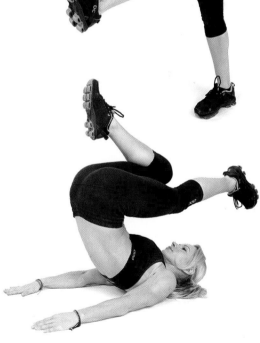

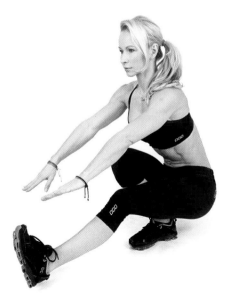

40. COMPETITION BURPEE TO ROCK-STAR JUMP

Starting position: Standing tall.

Movement: Bend at the knees and squat until you can place your palms on the ground. Using your arms for support, kick your legs behind you until you're in the upper push-up position. Do a push-up and then bring your legs forward so that you're once again in the low squat position. Jump, reaching back to touch your feet at the top.

Be careful to: Keep your form tight! There's a lot going on in this movement.

Notes: Repeat for the desired number of reps or the time allotted.

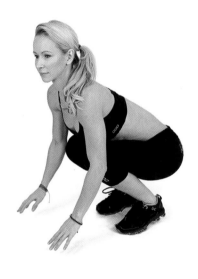

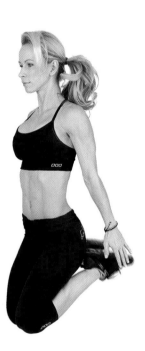

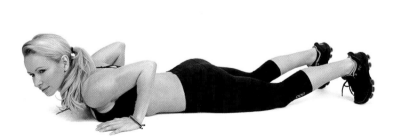

41. DIVE-BOMBER PUSH-UP

Starting position: Get in a push-up position and then transition to a downward dog position by shifting your weight back, so that if someone were viewing you from the side, your torso and legs would form an upside-down V.

Movement: Move your torso down between your hands, practically scraping the floor lightly with your nose, and then raise your torso so you're looking at the ceiling. Slowly resume the downward dog position.

Be careful to: Keep your muscles tight. If your form gets too loose on this move, your shoulders will suffer.

Notes: This is an advanced push-up that's great for shoulders and core!

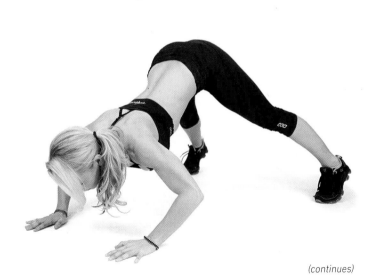

(continues)

Dive-Bomber Push-Up *(continued)*

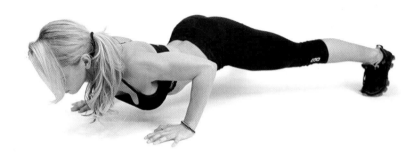

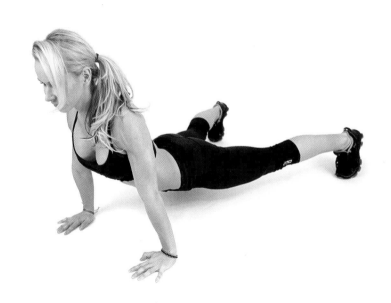

42. CRAB TOE TOUCH

Starting position: Get into crab-walk position: place your feet on the floor and your arms behind you so that your palms are flat on the floor. Your glutes should be lower than your shoulders and knees but not touching the floor.

Movement: Simultaneously raise one foot and reach up and over to touch it with the opposite side hand. Return to starting position. Do the same thing using the opposite hand and foot.

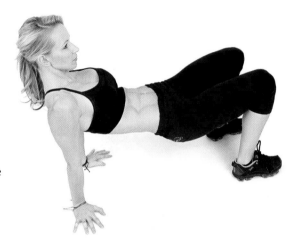

Be careful to: Keep your core tight or your form might falter.

Notes: Continue alternating for the desired number of reps or the time allotted.

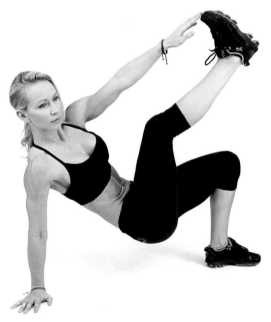

43. PIKE PRESS TO JUMP TUCK

Starting position: Plank position, feet a little wider apart than shoulder width. Push your hips up until your body looks like an upside-down V. Bend your elbows and bring your head as close to the floor as possible.

Movement: Push away from the floor with a lot of power to propel yourself into a squat position and then jump as high as you can, tucking your knees toward your chest.

Be careful to: Be stable in the lower squat before exploding upward.

Notes: You can use your arms for momentum on the jump.

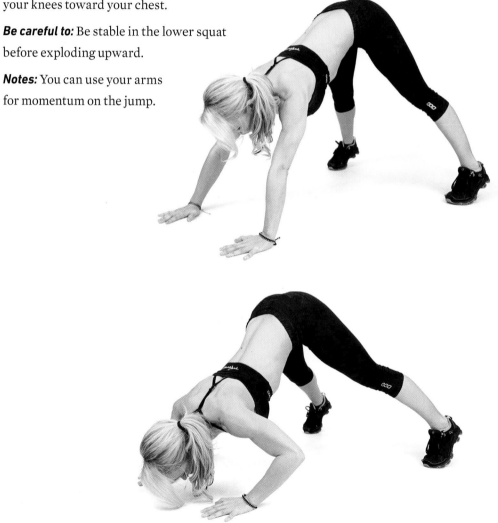

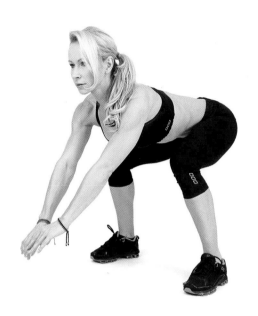

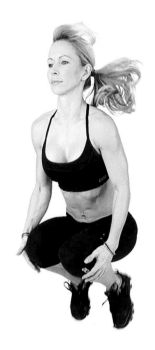

44. JUMP TUCK TO PISTOL

Starting position: Standing tall.

Movement: Jump as high as you can, tucking your knees close to your chest. As soon as you land back on your feet, shift your weight toward one leg, tense all of the muscles in the standing leg—including your glutes—and squat all the way down with the other leg and arms extended in front of you. Stand back up and repeat.

Be careful to: Go as deep as your strength and flexibility allow you to. Feel free to modify the pistol squat as shown on page 204.

Notes: If you stay consistent with your training, the depth of your pistol will gradually increase.

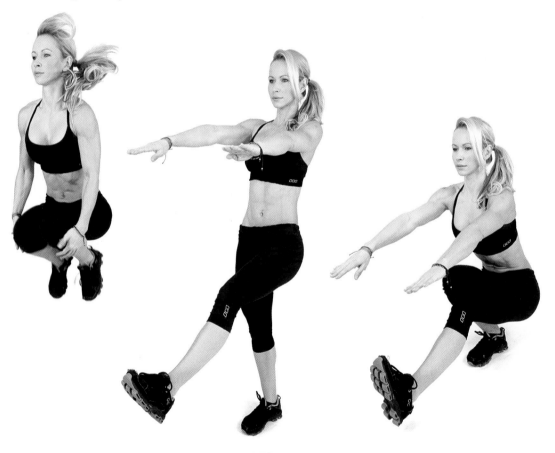

45. ONE-LEG DEADLIFT TO FRONT KICK

Starting position: Standing on one leg, tensing all the muscles in the standing leg.

Movement: Lean forward with your upper body, keeping your back straight, and extend the other leg behind you to make a T with your body. Reach to the ground with your fingertips and then use the power of your hips to stand back up and kick the back leg forward.

Be careful to: Make sure, when kicking forward, to flex your toes and kick through the heel, pushing your hips forward and squeezing your glutes.

Notes: When standing on one leg, tense all the muscles in that leg.

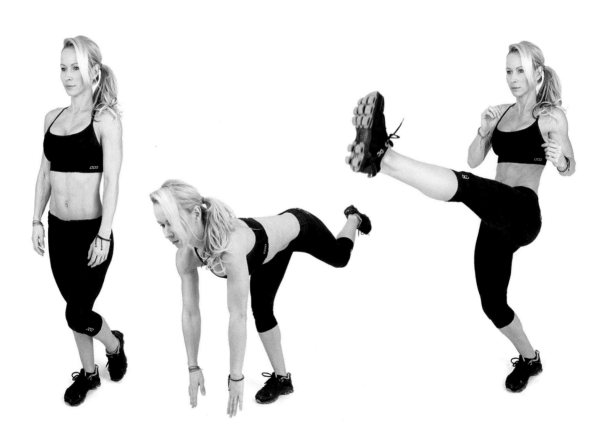

46. PUSH-UP TO ONE-LEG JUMP-UP

Starting position: A basic push-up position, with your hands directly underneath your shoulders and your body in a straight line. Make sure not to drop your hips or push them up. Tense all the muscles in your body, including your legs, glutes, and abs.

Movement: Bend your elbows to lower your torso until it nearly touches the ground. Press your torso back up to the starting position. From there, step forward with your right foot and push off that heel. Using your hips, drive up your left knee as you jump off your right leg. Land on the ball of your right foot and then resume plank. Do the same number of reps for each side.

Be careful to: Keep your elbows from flaring out during the push-up.

Notes: Continue alternating for the desired number of reps or the time allotted.

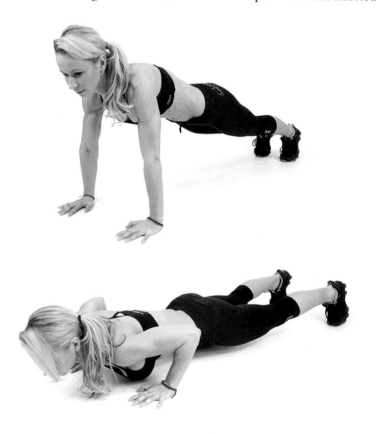

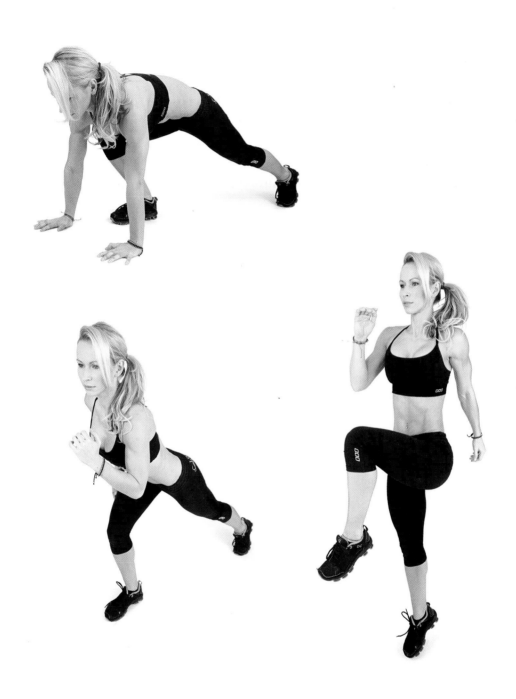

47. ONE-ARM PRESS-UP

Starting position: Lie down on your belly and place one hand directly under your shoulder with your elbow pointing behind you. Keep your legs a little bit wider apart and place the other hand on your thigh or else make a fist and place it on your lower back—whatever is more comfortable for you but gets your other hand out of the way.

Movement: Push off the floor with your hand until your arm is fully extended and your abs are off the ground. Do not shrug your shoulder. Now dig your toes into the ground and push your hips up and back to create an upside-down V with your body in the pike position. Lift your tailbone up and press your chest toward your thighs. Try your best to keep your knees locked. Reverse the movement and bring your body down to the ground.

Be careful to: Keep your knees slightly bent if you're not flexible enough yet to do this without strain. You can also place both hands on the ground if using one hand is too difficult.

Notes: Always make sure to do the same number of reps on each arm.

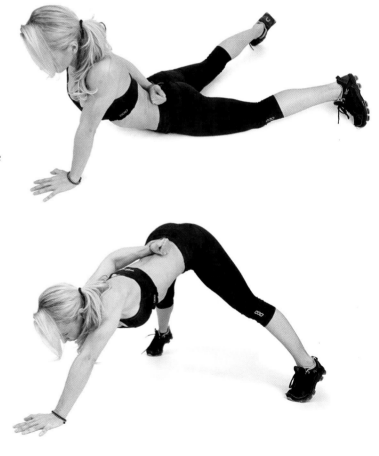

48. TWISTED PUSH-UP TOE TOUCH

Starting position: Get into crab-walk position; place your feet on the floor and your arms behind you so that your palms are flat on the floor. Your glutes should be lower than your shoulders and knees but not touching the floor.

Movement: Lift your left foot and right hand off the ground, and twisting your body toward your left, bring the right foot under your left knee and flip over into a plank. Keep that left foot off the ground for greater challenge if you want and do a push-up. Reverse the movement to get back into the crab-walk position, lift the right leg up and touch your toes with your left hand.

Be careful to: Do not shrug your shoulders in the starting position. Keep them away from your ears.

Notes: Repeat for the prescribed amount of reps and then switch sides. You can make the push-up easier by going onto your knees or just bending your elbows only as much as your strength allows you to. You'll be able to get closer to the ground if you stay consistent with your training.

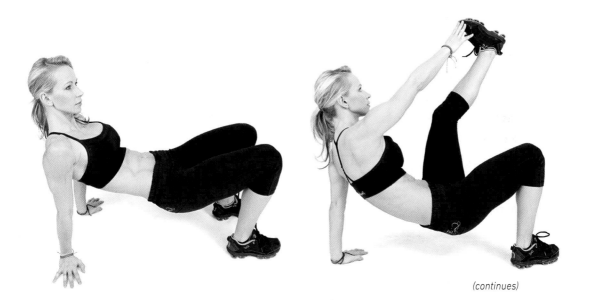

(continues)

Twisted Push-Up Toe Touch (continued)

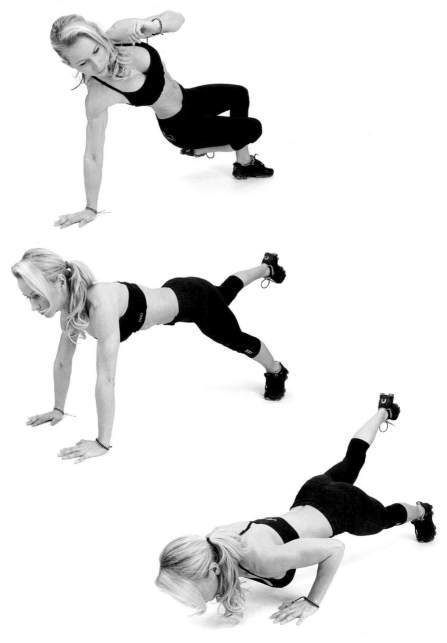

49. SUMO SQUAT LEG LIFT

Starting position: Standing tall, feet wide apart, toes pointing slightly outward.

Movement: Bend your knees and push your hips back until your thighs are parallel to the ground. Extend your knees to straighten up, and as you reach the upright position, shift your weight immediately toward one leg and lift the other leg out to the side.

Be careful to: Keep your stance nice and wide. These are called sumo squats for a reason.

Notes: Repeat by alternating legs on each squat.

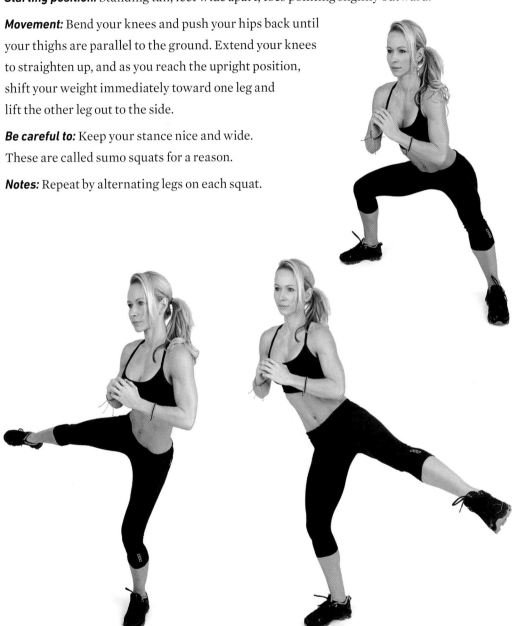

50. ROCK-STAR JUMP

Starting position: Standing tall.

Movement: Jump! As your feet reach your glutes, reach back with your hands and touch them.

Be careful to: The more movement you generate, the more calories you'll burn.

Notes: Once you land, repeat for the desired number of reps or the time allotted.

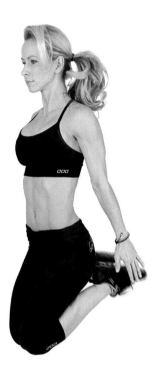

When Should You Work Out?

One of the great things about my workouts is that you can do them anywhere, anytime, and they still take only 15 minutes. However, I'm a big believer in training in the morning, and it has to do with more than personal preference.

Waking up early to train will not only help you get in better shape but will also make preparation for the whole day much easier. Because you need to get ready and your muscles need to be warmed up before an actual workout, you naturally will get up even earlier and have time to enjoy a nice fresh-brewed cup of coffee and even prepare your own meal, which is as important as the workout. Eating a healthy breakfast and lunch not only will help you build healthy habits but will also prevent you from eating junk food during the day.

When you start working out in the mornings, you're going to feel more energized and alert for the rest of the day. Because we are living in a fast-paced world, full of technology and distractions, it is extremely hard to stay focused, calm, and organized. You'll be able to use your organized mind to set health and fitness goals and focus on achieving them. When you wake up early in the morning you naturally get more done throughout the day, and feel more accomplished and happy. As Benjamin Franklin once said: "Early to bed and early to rise, makes a [person] healthy, wealthy, and wise." You can also burn more calories when you work out in the morning, as your metabolism works much faster and better and will help keep your weight more under control.

Exercise can help clear your mind. Any type of workout will stimulate blood circulation and will naturally increase blood flow in your brain. More blood means more energy and oxygen, which makes your brain perform better. When you're working out, concentrate on something positive. It will give you more energy and stamina and you will feel more centered and empowered.

Exercising in the morning boosts endorphins in the brain, which will elevate your mood and offer you physical and mental gratification for the rest of the day. Endorphins also trigger a positive feeling in the body. For example, the feeling that follows a run or workout is often described as euphoric. Having endorphin boosts on a daily basis will help you reduce stress, fight off any feelings of anxiety and depression, improve your sleep and metabolism, and definitely boost your self-esteem. What's more, you will be looking fit and healthy. Working out in the mornings will help you get a positive outlook on life on every level.

Mother Nature's Pre-workout

Many of us reach for a cup of coffee or tea first thing in the morning. Did you know that caffeine is also a good thing to have right before a workout? Not only does caffeine act as a mild stimulant, providing the typical buzz most of us are used to, it actually qualifies as a legal performance enhancer when used by athletes for workouts and competitions. According to studies done at McMaster University in Canada, caffeine temporarily increases the efficiency of our muscles, providing greater endurance and power. Mark Tarnopolsky, a competitive triathlete who also headed these various studies on exercise and caffeine, is convinced that caffeine substantially improves athletic performance.

Caffeine also provides a small but significant amount of pain relief during exercise, enabling us to potentially work past our normal stopping points when training for strength and endurance. According to a study published in *Nutrition and Metabolism*, caffeine allowed the participants of a recent study to maintain higher levels of intensity during a workout. The researchers, echoing the McMaster study, noted that "the performance enhancing effects of caffeine are very clear."

Try drinking four ounces of coffee or the equivalent in tea (tea has less caffeine per cup than coffee) an hour before a workout. Just don't reach for something loaded with calories like the dessert drinks you find at many coffee shops. Keep it simple.

Should You Train When You're Sick?

If you think you're coming down with the flu or if someone close to you has the flu—for example, a spouse or a child—do not, I repeat, *do not* try to blast your way through one of my intense 15-minute workouts.

While exercise supports the immune system, intense exercise while ill or on the verge of illness has been shown to be detrimental to our immune system's response to viruses such as the flu. It can actually make the symptoms of the cold and flu more severe.

It can also increase the duration of the illness. Much research seems to suggest that the level of stress an intense workout puts on our bodies keeps it from effectively focusing on fighting the flu bug. Our immune defenses are down for the count when we've exhausted ourselves through strenuous exercise.

What you can do and ought to do if you feel a seasonal illness coming on is exercise at a moderate, even gentle pace. A long walk or a slow, short jog might be just the ticket to keeping your body in battle mode against the flu. While studies seem pretty clear that intense exercise should be avoided right before or during the onset of illness because of the body is in a temporarily weakened state of immunity, the same studies also indicate that moderate exercise does in fact *boost* the immune system.

What If You Start Feeling Tired?

Fatigue is usually a combination of factors. For example, an argument with your boss may create stress that, in turn, causes you to binge on ice cream and chips instead of that kale salad you prepared the night before. Not only are you mentally fatigued by the argument but you made a poor food choice, which left you more tired. *Recognizing* the cause of fatigue is the key to getting back on track. Here are four common causes of fatigue:

(continues)

1. *Not drinking enough water throughout the day.* This is an incredibly common cause of fatigue and sluggishness. Hydration is vital for our well-being.
2. *Too few healthy nutrients, too much sugar.* Fruits and vegetables are fatigue fighters, as are whole grains and sources of lean protein. Too much sugar, on the other hand, causes a brief, short-lived spike in energy followed by a crash.
3. *Mental fatigue.* Sometimes the most beneficial thing to do to fight fatigue, mental or otherwise, is to exercise, but getting past that initial hurdle when you're tired can seem like an impossible task. Meditation provides focus and acts as a dimmer switch to all the senseless chatter and anxiety that can sometimes overwhelm us.
4. *Not enough rest!* Lack of sleep is a guaranteed method of turning yourself into a zombie.

CHAPTER 10

The Great Balancing Act: Fitness and Your Life

Fitness and well-being are not just about diet and exercise, although you can't be fit without working out and eating well. When the next workout or meal ends, everything you do still affects your body in some way. This is an extreme example, but if you work out, eat a healthy meal, and then light up a cigarette, you're undoing the positive things you just did. Likewise, if you sleep for only two hours the night after a hard workout and a nutritious dinner, you're not tying it all together in a way that will lead to lasting success. It's kind of pointless to be Arnold Schwarzenegger during your workout and Jabba the Hutt the rest of the time. Your joints and muscles are miraculous creations, but they're as vulnerable to misuse as they are to no use at all.

Fitness isn't just about the body, either; it's about the mind too. After working out intensely, you must unwind. Relaxation and rejuvenation are just as important as hard work. Without balance, no one achieves his or her desired results. You're simply not in balance without a proper recovery from my 15-minute workouts.

So what is proper recovery? Is it trying to stretch to your toes and then taking a selfie of you dripping your colored Gatorade sweat? Nah. Proper recovery entails certain basics: sleep, waking relaxation, nutrition, hydration, and some sort of flexibility training—something a little more serious than crossing your arms over your body twice. However, recovery *can* include much more than the basics: everything from acupuncture, massage therapy, and aromatherapy to meditation and electronic muscle stimulation. Some people get so far into this that they sit in infrared saunas and float in sensory deprivation tanks. Regardless of the technique, the basics are a must—even if the stretching consists of basic static stretches post-workout and even if the relaxation is simply reading a good book.

Ten Mental Activities for Recovery

There are plenty of relaxing activities, and all you need is to dedicate 15 minutes a day for yourself to recharge. If you don't take care of yourself, who will?

1. *Read a nice book.* The pages can actually take you to a new place. Get lost in a story other than your own.
2. *Meditate.* Calm your mind, and your body will tell you what's hurting or needs to be relaxed. This is the ultimate way to find out what you really think and feel.
3. *Listen to music.* Blast it, play it softly, sing along, cry, dance, whatever you want. Whatever gets you relaxed or feeling better—do it.
4. *Play a musical instrument.* Unless you suck. Then play it away from me.
5. *Decorate your home.* Tidy up the place. Make it an oasis rather than a stressful reminder of another chore you have to do.
6. *Play with your pet (or a child).* Remember how to have fun. Your pet's or child's happiness will quickly rub off on you.
7. *Spend quality time with a loved one.* Happiness is better when shared. Do something new and make a memory.
8. *Take a bubble bath or jump into a Jacuzzi.* Do I even need to say why? Mmmmm, sweet relaxation.

9. *Light some candles.* Daydream about something positive. Mind over matter. What you believe becomes your reality.

10. *Do some gardening.* It not only looks good, but if you grow your own food, it can save you money! Talk about a win-win.

It's easy to overlook something as simple as stretching because it's not as transformative or as fun as working out. But if you want to stay flexible as you age, it's a must. Stretching and proper recovery as a whole play a major role in injury prevention. They even promote healthy aging by maintaining muscle tone and decreasing free-radical damage within the body and on the skin. Less damage of this sort means your arms, butt, and face are less saggy and baggy. Don't get me wrong—our faces will still wrinkle, and no plastic surgery can yank your face back enough to make you look you're 20 years old if you're 39. (And who would want that, anyway? Remember how overwhelming life seemed when you were 20?) But the things you can do to keep your body strong and flexible are incredible. I've seen older people performing unbelievable athletic feats and having a blast in their pain-free bodies. To me the goal is not just length of life but also quality of life.

You Did Your 15-Minute Workout. Great! Now What?

Getting stronger, fitter, and leaner is a combination of exposing your body to high-stress activity, such as one of my workouts, and then recovering from it. The faster you can recover, the better your results. If you don't recover adequately from the stress that working out has imposed on your body, you'll get tired and your body will stop making gains.

Don't forget to stretch after the workout ends. This is super-important for proper recovery, and it can help reduce or prevent the muscle soreness that often kicks in 48 hours or so after a workout. A recent study in the *Journal of Athletic Training* reported a 5 percent decrease in delayed-onset muscle soreness (DOMS) when athletes used static stretching immediately after a workout. Although they didn't look at the effects, the authors encouraged dynamic stretches and low-intensity movement within one to three days after an intense workout to minimize DOMS. The athletes reported that the static stretches decreased the transient soreness after the onset of DOMS.

Along with stretching, I love using a foam roller after I work out. This cylindrical piece of hard foam can be rolled over your muscles against the pressure of your own body weight. Foam rolling works best on the lower extremities such as the glutes, calves, quads, and hamstrings. It's also highly effective along the iliotibial (IT) band running along the sides of the upper legs. Tight IT bands contribute to a lot of pain and discomfort in other areas such as the knees for athletes and active people alike. Regardless of which tissues you're targeting, the foam roller is a great do-it-yourself tool for releasing knotted trigger points. Left unaddressed, knots can cause pain, muscular imbalances, and mobility issues.

As with any deep-tissue massage technique, foam rolling can hurt sometimes. Don't go crazy until tears stream down your face, but don't go too easy on yourself either. The more tight and painful an area feels, the more you need to address it. Sometimes you need to feel some pain before you can feel better.

Having stretched and used the foam roller after your workout, you'll decide what, if anything, to eat or drink. Along with sleep, diet is the most critical factor in workout recovery. After an intense session, your body may be pretty depleted, so it's natural to want to refuel. But don't reach for a bag of chips or a slice of pizza, even if it's convenient and seems appealing. Focus on eating real food, not junk food. Eat fruits, vegetables, and lean meats and avoid eating too much salt and sugar. Foods high in sugar, trans fats, and preservatives slow you down and do little to help you become fit and strong.

Your body needs protein in particular to build muscle. If you don't give your body protein within a reasonable amount of time after working out, you start losing some of the potential of muscle synthesis and growth. According to a prominent researcher at the University of Texas, once protein is consumed, there is a three-hour window of protein synthesis, with a peak between 45 and 90 minutes after consumption.

Research suggests that the sooner you can consume protein, especially the amino acid leucine, the more efficiently post-workout protein synthesis will occur. This includes consuming protein *before* your workout so the pieces are in place to promote muscle growth during the workout and not just afterward.

Everyone's a little different, though. Personally, I can't eat anything solid for at least an hour after my workout. Luckily for me, liquid protein works better than whole-food protein after a workout. It is more readily available to be used by the muscles that need it, rather than having to go through the digestion process before it can be absorbed by your body. Even after a workout, your muscles are still working, and redirecting blood flow to the gut isn't necessarily going to take precedence. As a result the meal can just sort of sit in your stomach. This is probably why a lot of people don't like to eat after a good workout.

The Rest of Your Day

For the rest of your day, I want you to focus on *recovery*. Beyond the period immediately after your workout, numerous strategies can enhance recovery. Just because the workout is over doesn't mean you can't stay active. Try to fit some light physical activities into your schedule, especially those that include lots of flexibility work: stretching, an easy yoga workout, a bike ride, or a nice long walk with your dog—anything that gets you off the couch. It's important to move about and burn calories throughout the day, not just for 15 minutes.

Enjoying your rest periods means doing things that make you feel good. You don't always have to meditate with your legs crossed and eyes closed. Reading a book, listening to music, playing with your dog, or playing a guitar for at least 15 minutes can offer the same feelings of relaxation and escape. Chores, work, and everyday stress easily overwhelm us, and we sometimes forget to find a little bit of time for ourselves. It's always the little things that make us happy and make life worth living.

The body, mind, and soul are closely connected, so any kind of stress experienced outside of your workouts can influence your health and energy levels. We have to focus not only on physical recovery but also on mental and emotional healing. Stress from work, relationships, money, or your environment can have a negative impact on your immune system. If your cortisol levels are always up due to chronic anxiety and stress, your exercise performance will suffer and so will your results. Again, a body under so much stress needs sufficient recovery before you can expect any improvement.

The Fluids Factor

Drinking plenty of fluids is vital for fitness and well-being. We are, after all, mostly water. Drinking plenty of water is important before workouts as well as after workouts. Sports drinks are OK only during intense exercise because they replenish vital electrolytes, of which the most important is sodium. Pickle juice, believe it or not, is a great recovery/replenishment alternative. However, day to day, when you're not exercising, water is the perfect choice. Some people do not like plain water because it's, well, plain! So add some fruit slices. I like to add slices of strawberries and lemons.

Sleep

The human body secretes most of its growth hormone (GH) in two windows: after a hard workout and during sleep. GH values are highest first thing in the morning. As you can see, if you make time to work out but not to sleep, you're shooting yourself in the foot. In fact, missing sleep is worse than missing a workout, in my opinion. Naps are a good idea when you fail to sleep for eight hours. Remember, many people around the world enjoy daily siestas! If you're having trouble falling asleep at night, I recommend taking a warm bath before bedtime. Another practice I highly recommend is going to sleep and waking up at the same time every day. Increasing sleep time on the weekend, for example, can alter your body's natural cortisol release pattern, actually increasing it. So you can't expect to sleep poorly all week and then make up for it on the weekend. The body doesn't work that way.

Stretching

Stretching is vitally important. I'm a strong believer in the mind–body connection, and as part of that connection, I believe you have to stretch every day to remain flexible rather than becoming chronically stiff. While it's not necessary to be as flexible as a ballerina or circus acrobat, try stretching for 15 to 20 minutes after a workout or before going to bed. Otherwise you can even stretch while you're watching television! Regardless of when I stretch, I achieve enhanced flexibility and decreased soreness by holding the stretch for 3 to 5 minutes rather than for 30 seconds, which is the standard recommendation. However, if I have only 30 seconds for a short stretch, I use it and I do it. Every moment counts!

Massage

Massaging your muscles not only soothes aches and pains but also helps increase circulation, which aids in recovery. A review in the journal *Sports Medicine* reported that various types of massage altered neural excitability, parasympathetic activity, and cortisol levels; decreased anxiety; and improved mood. Not all types of massage supported all of these results, but there were more positive outcomes than negative. Two studies in particular reported reduced muscle soreness with massage two hours postexercise, purportedly due to increased microcirculation of blood and lymph.

As with stretching, massage increases mobility and loosens up tight spots in our bodies, such as between our shoulder blades and along our IT band on the outside of our thighs.

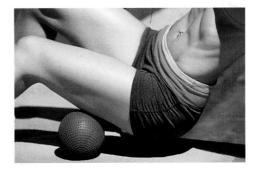

Some of us consider a massage relaxing but not necessarily therapeutic. Sure, it may feel good, but its benefits are often judged in the same way as is a manicure or a trip to the salon. Yet a proper massage done by a professional has numerous benefits for our physical bodies as well as our mental and emotional well-being.

Massage therapy can be helpful in managing pain, especially back pain, without the use of medications. According Daniel C. Cherkin, PhD, senior investigator at Group Health Research Institute, who headed a 2011 study published in the *Annals of Internal Medicine*, proper massage can be as effective in helping manage back pain as yoga, acupuncture, and painkillers. Massage can also help counter the effects of headaches caused by tension or migraines, labor pains, and certain types of arthritis.

If you've ever dozed off on the massage table, there's a reason for it. Massage improves our sleep. In fact, some studies indicate that massage therapy increases our delta waves, important brain waves associated with deep sleep.

Massage therapy is one effective way to increase circulation around our sore muscles and aid in the recovery process. Massage therapy also helps with muscles that tend to tighten up over time, such as the back and outer legs. Tight muscles not only cause pain but can also lead to injury. Our muscles should be strong and sexy, not rigid and stiff. Massage, along with stretching and mobility work, is a great way to keep our muscles supple. Part of the reason a massage feels so relaxing is because, physiologically speaking, it is!

Meditation

Various academic studies have shown that meditation is perhaps the best way to train the mind and provide it with relief from daily stress and anxiety. Meditation also allows us to focus on the important aspects of our lives rather than fixating on things of lesser importance, such as bad traffic or workplace drama. We don't necessarily have to follow a specific religion or spiritual path to gain the benefits for meditation, either, though it's perfectly fine if you do. In fact, Sam Harris, a well-known neuroscientist, is a staunch atheist who also happens to be a dedicated practitioner of meditation.

Here are four reasons to make meditation a part of your fitness routine:

Focus. Meditation allows for greater concentration in our lives. A recent study out of the University of California, Santa Barbara, demonstrated that meditation decreased wandering, aimless thoughts and improved memory, especially when associated with specific tasks such as studying or learning a new skill.

It's good for your body too. Aside from benefiting our minds, meditation can be important for our physical health. Now research suggests that consistent meditation may reduce the risk of heart attack and stroke by 48 percent compared with those who do not meditate.

Increased brain function. Researchers at the University of California, Los Angeles, found a greater increase in the cerebral cortex in participants who meditated. Growth in this specific area of the brain also indicates that those who consistently meditate may be able to process information at a faster rate than those who do not.

Stress! More than anything else, meditation is a healthy way to manage stress. Done correctly and consistently, meditation can practically breathe away the daily worries that bother you during the day and keep you up at night.

There are a variety of ways to meditate. Some people chant, some pray, some simply breathe while focusing on their diaphragm. Find a method that suits your lifestyle, temperament, and beliefs. Mindfulness meditation is increasingly popular and relatively simple, but it's not the only method out there. Like diet and exercise, meditation is not always easy, but it may very well be worth it.

Surviving Your Ugly Days

"Ugly days" affect most people but especially women. If you're human, there's a 99.9 percent chance that you've already experienced an ugly day. I'm sure you'll relate when I describe exactly what an ugly day is. You find yourself in front of a mirror nitpicking everything about the way you look. You're feeling too fat or too skinny or maybe there's something about your face you don't like. You're just not feeling pretty, and it's bringing you down.

You think there's something wrong with you and you may even feel worthless. Suddenly it's starting to make sense that if you were not so fat, ugly, or skinny, or if

(continues)

you didn't have that big nose, you'd be happy. That's when everything can go really wrong. People start to obsess about the way they look, and before they know it, they develop body image, eating, and anxiety disorders.

That's why it's important that we deal with ugly days in a healthy way and take them for what they are—only ugly days. I love this Audrey Hepburn quote: "Happy girls are the prettiest girls." This simple sentence conveys so much wisdom and truth. If you think about it, have you ever been concerned about the way you look when you were laughing with your friends or playing with your kids or participating in a sport you love? Of course not. During the happiest moments of our lives, we all are the most beautiful and confident people in the world.

This is my own quote: "Happiness is confidence without effort." Confidence is what makes people charismatic and attractive, and that's why you have to believe in yourself and be proud of who you are, right? Well, that can take a conscious effort at times, but when you're happy, you're already confident and charismatic by default.

So the next time you have an ugly day, realize there is nothing wrong with *you*. Maybe you're bored. Maybe you don't like your current job. You are beautiful; you're just not having fun for whatever reason. Figure out the reason and see what you can do to fix that. Just remember that all you are experiencing is nothing more than an ugly day, and there are so many happy days to come.

Saving Your Back

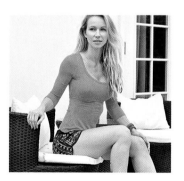

Unfortunately, lower back pain is widespread these days, affecting about 80 percent of the people in the United States at one point or another. Our increasingly sedentary lives at work and home don't help. Simply put, we sit way too much, and poor posture and a limited range of motion often result. Sitting places undue stress on our hamstrings and hip flexors, and consequently on our lower back, neck, and hips.

Aches and Pains

Tweaks and strains are common enough when working out, but often a minor ache can turn into a major nuisance if left unaddressed. Overuse injuries can occur for a variety of reasons, including lack of recovery, poor sleep, and fatigue. Fatigue leads to bad form, and bad form can cause injury.

Bad posture is another factor that puts unnecessary stress on the body over time. This leads to muscular and skeletal imbalances that can lead to overuse injuries. Here are three common overuse injuries and how to help manage and, more important, prevent them.

1. *Neck strain.* If you sit at a desk for extended periods of time at work or at home, you've more than likely experienced a dull to sharp ache at the back of your neck. This is caused by an unnatural forward tilt that develops in front of computer screens. It's important not to look down constantly while working, but rather to look straight ahead with proper posture—shoulders back and relaxed in the same manner as when standing. Neck strain is often made worse when you don't maintain a neutral neck position when working out. Whether you're doing squats or push-ups, always look straight ahead. This will help maintain the natural curvature of your spine. Looking up or down places an unnatural amount of stress on the vertebrae in your neck, which can lead to pain or injury.

2. *Knee pain.* Knee pain is a common overuse injury, and in most cases, it's avoidable. Proper form when performing exercises such as squats, burpees, and lunges goes a long way toward saving your knees. First and foremost, your knees should never bend or buckle inward from any type of squat-based movement; they should always extend slightly outward. Always drive from your heels, not your toes or the front of the foot, as you're pushing up. This allows the force to be properly distributed to your muscles and reduces the stress on your knees.

3. *Lower back pain.* Perhaps the most common overuse injury, lower back pain, can nag us for days if not years due to bad posture when sitting and standing.

(continues)

It's also made worse from a weak, unbalanced core. Rounding the lower back when working out is a major cause of pain and injury. Always maintain a neutral or arched back, especially when doing exercises such as kettlebell swings, squats, and deadlifts. Also, consistently stretching your glutes, hip flexors, and hamstrings loosens up the lower back and reduces the amount of stress placed on it from bad posture and form.

At some point, many people experience a dull, nagging ache in their lower back or even a sudden sharp pain while lifting or while playing sports. They also spend hours at a time slumping in chairs or standing with bad posture, adding more stress to their already sore lumbar spine region.

One reason I'm a big fan of body weight exercises is that they take less toll on the lower back than bodybuilding and CrossFit. Weight training is way better than being sedentary, but safe lifting for the long haul requires correct form. Unless you train with a highly knowledgeable personal trainer, what are the odds you're using correct form? Most people who don't have proper guidance and coaching are doing something wrong on nearly every exercise. It may be only a minor thing, like your knee coming out half an inch farther than your toes on your squats, but doing thousands of reps over time with compromised form adds up to and makes for some serious wear. Fortunately, the images in this book offer all the guidance you need.

So many people who lift weights their whole life need disc surgery in their forties and beyond. And many of them are never the same physically after such problems strike. The human spine is miraculous: It has to be strong enough to support an entire body yet flexible enough to allow us to bend, twist, and lift things day in, day out for decade upon decade. Much of the structural stability comes from our vertebrae, and much of our flexibility comes from the discs in between them. Over time those discs can be damaged, and eventually they can bulge and even herniate or rupture, leading in most cases to pain and a loss of mobility. Nerves running along our spinal column control many of our most basic and important movements, and it doesn't take much to damage those nerves.

I'm not saying that training with only your body weight eliminates the possibilityof a back injury. I had trouble with a bulging disc a few years ago, but I attribute that mostly to having scoliosis. Moreover, I was able to address the problem without surgery. But I would argue that body weight exercises are safer for your back than lifting weights. In the squat rack or power rack, lifters can let their ego get the better of them and lift more weight than their body is equipped to handle. You'd be hardpressed to place yourself at such risk by doing too many push-ups or burpees.

OK, you're probably thinking. *So how do I stretch my lower back?* That's a trick question, actually. Let me explain. A stiff lower back is really the result of tight hamstrings, hip flexors, and/or glutes. These three large muscle groups are anchored to the lower back. When they tighten, they pull chronically and awkwardly on the lower back, causing tightness, soreness, or worse, muscle spasms.

So you need to take a broader view of back health. Think of your abdominal and lower-back muscles as the body's natural back brace. The stronger they become, the healthier your back. Planks and leg raises are a fantastic way to quickly and efficiently build core strength. Along with strengthening your abdominal muscles, strengthen your lower back. Your spinal erectors are those long muscles that travel along your spine, and the best body weight exercises for strengthening them are squats and deadlifts. You can isolate your back more with exercises such as the Superman, but I always prefer multijoint functional exercises that mimic more of a natural movement. After all, the human body naturally works as a unit.

Never brush aside back pain if it lingers or if the pain is sudden and sharp. Either could be a sign of a herniated disc or of some other serious injury. Please see a doctor as soon as possible if there is any tingling or numbness in your back, legs, or elsewhere. A lot of chiropractors now use the active release technique (ART)—which is basically passive or assisted stretching while the practitioner pushes through the tight muscle or knot—rather than spinal adjustments because it's the tight muscles that pull the spine and hips out of alignment. ART is amazing and painful all at the same time, especially on the hamstrings and glutes, those super-tight spots that often lead to lower back pain. Once a muscle is loosened up, the spine often returns to functioning normally!

Six Physical Activities for Recovery

Exerting energy from your body takes a lot of the stress from your mind. By taking advantage of the following healing activities, you can recover from both physical and mental stress.

1. *Do some yoga.* Handstands or just child's pose. I'm gonna stick with child's pose.

2. *Stretch your body.* Mmmm, feel the burn. The tighter your muscles, the less relaxed you are. Really loosen 'em up.

3. *Sweat it out, baby.* Do some cardio and let the stress drip away.

4. *Take a long walk with your dog.* Because who doesn't love puppies? ::adopts 600::

5. *Go for a swim.* Maybe you're not Michael Phelps, but we won't judge you for doing the dog paddle. Just keep swimming . . . and swimming.

6. *Dance.* Do it for fun, not for performance. Let the music take you over. Don't worry, no one's watching. (They will be, though, because this video of you dancing is so going on Facebook.)

Bibliography

Adam, T. C., and E. S. Epel. "Stress, Eating and the Reward System." *Physiology and Behavior* 91, no. 4 (2007): 449–458.

Alessio, H. M., A. H. Goldfarb, and G. Cao. "Exercise-Induced Oxidative Stress Before and After Vitamin C Supplementation." *International Journal of Sport Nutrition* 7, no. 1 (1997): 1–9.

Baekeland, F., and R. Lasky. "Exercise and Sleep Patterns in College Athletes." *Perceptual and Motor Skills* 23, no. 3 (1966): 1203–1207.

Benson, H., L. Kagan, and B. Kessel. *Mind over Menopause: The Complete Mind/Body Approach to Coping with Menopause.* Atria, 2004.

Cutt, H., B. Giles-Corti, M. Knuiman, and V. Burke. "Dog Ownership, Health and Physical Activity: A Critical Review of the Literature." *Health Place* 13, no. 1 (2007): 261–272.

Dorrens, J., and M. J. Rennie. "Effects of Ageing and Human Whole Body and Muscle Protein Turnover." *Scandinavian Journal of Medicine and Science in Sports* 13, no. 1 (2003): 26–33.

Egoscue, P., and R. Gittines. *Pain Free: A Revolutionary Method for Stopping Chronic Pain.* Bantam, 2000.

Freimuth, M., S. Moniz, and S. R. Kim. "Clarifying Exercise Addiction: Differential Diagnosis, Co-Occurring Disorders, and Phases of Addiction." *International Journal of Environmental Research and Public Health* 8, no. 10 (2011): 4069–4081.

Goldfarb, A. H., and A. Z. Jamurtas. "Beta-Endorphin Response to Exercise. An Update." *Sports Medicine* 24, no. 1 (1997): 8–16.

Harris, A. H., R. Cronkite, and R. Moos. "Physical Activity, Exercise Coping, and Depression in a 10-Year Cohort Study of Depressed Patients." *Journal of Affective Disorders* 93, no. 1–3 (2006): 79–85.

Larsson, L., G. Grimby, and J. Karlsson. "Muscle Strength and Speed of Movement in Relation to Age and Muscle Morphology." *Journal of Applied Physiology: Respiratory, Environmental, and Exercise Physiology* 46, no. 3 (1979): 451–456.

Lindle, R. S., E. J. Metter, N. A. Lynch, et al. "Age and Gender Comparisons of Muscle Strength in 654 Women and Men Aged 20–93 Yr." *Journal of Applied Physiology* 83, no. 5 (1997): 1581–1587.

Stillar, A. "The Effects of Stress on Eating Patterns and the Effects of Stress and Attachment on Eating Behavior and Food Preference in Stress Under-Eaters and Stress-Eaters." Master's thesis. Laurentian University, Sudbury, Ontario, Canada, 2015.

Thacker, S. B., J. Gilchrist, D. F. Stroup, and C. D. Kimsey Jr. "The Impact of Stretching on Sports Injury Risk: A Systematic Review of the Literature." *Medicine and Science in Sports and Exercise* 36, no. 3 (2004): 371–378.

Torres, S. J., and C. A. Nowson. "Relationship Between Stress, Eating Behavior, and Obesity." *Nutrition* 23, no. 11–12 (2007): 887–894.

Villeneuve, P. J., H. I. Morrison, C. L. Craig, and D. E. Schaubel. "Physical Activity, Physical Fitness, and Risk of Dying." *Epidemiology* 9, no. 6 (1998): 626–631.

Weerapong, P., P. A. Hume, and G. S. Kolt. "The Mechanisms of Massage and Effects on Performance, Muscle Recovery and Injury Prevention." *Sports Medicine* 35, no. 3 (2005): 235–256.

Weller, I., and P. Corey. "The Impact of Excluding Non-Leisure Energy Expenditure on the Relation Between Physical Activity and Mortality in Women." *Epidemiology* 9, no. 6 (1998): 632–635.

Wells, D. L. "Domestic Dogs and Human Health: An Overview." *British Journal of Health Psychology* 12, pt. 1 (2007): 145–156.

Zellner, D. A., S. Loaiza, Z. Gonzalez, et al. "Food Selection Changes Under Stress." *Physiology and Behavior* 87, no. 4 (2006): 789–793.

Acknowledgments

I would like to thank everyone who made this book possible, starting with my co-author, Bodybuilding.com editor in chief Jeff O'Connell, who helped give voice to both my personal story and my fitness plan. My manager, Will Hobbs of Key Priority Management, and Jeff's literary agent, Marc Gerald of the Agency Group, presented our idea for *15 Minutes to Fit* to publishers, a team effort for which I am very grateful.

Fortunately for us, the book project landed in the very capable hands of Megan Newman, publisher of Avery, an imprint of Penguin Random House. Our editor, Gigi Campo, helped shape the manuscript into what you're holding in your hands. (We couldn't have done it without you, Gigi!) I'm also indebted to Caroline Sutton, editor in chief; Lindsay Gordon, publicity and marketing director; Anne Kosmoski, publicist; Ally Bruschi, publicity assistant; and Roshe Anderson, marketing coordinator. A big THANK-YOU to everyone at Avery for believing in me and helping us.

I also would like to thank Ashley A. Herda, PhD, CSCS*D, a lecturer and academic program associate in the Department of Health, Sport, and Exercise Sciences at the University of Kansas (Edwards), for being our science consultant on the project; and Tiffiny Trentalange for her transcription services. Ashley Erin Dean, who helps run my website, also deserves a high five.

I really want to give a big shout-out to everyone who has watched my videos and visited my website over the years. I wish I could give all of you a giant Z hug in person for your support, but this note will have to do for now. Your feedback and support over the years have been immensely helpful, and I appreciate it more than words can express.

And last but not least, I'd like to thank my boyfriend, Jesse Heer, who's been with me through the toughest times of my life and fought many of my battles for me when I didn't have the strength. It wouldn't have been possible without you.

Index